Therapeutic Interventions for the Person with Dementia

Therapeutic Interventions for the Person with Dementia

Ellen D. Taira
Editor

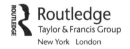

Routledge
Taylor & Francis Group
New York   London

Therapeutic Interventions for the Person with Dementia has also been published as *Physical & Occupational Therapy in Geriatrics*, Volume 4, Number 3, Spring 1986.

First published 1986 by
The Haworth Press, Inc., 28 East 22 Street, New York, NY 10010-6194
EUROSPAN/Haworth, 3 Henrietta Street, London WC2E 8LU England

This edition published 2014 by Routledge

Routledge
Taylor & Francis Group
711 Third Avenue
New York, NY 10017

Routledge
Taylor & Francis Group
2 Park Square, Milton Park
Abingdon, Oxon OX14 4RN

Routledge is an imprint of the Taylor & Francis Group, an informa business

Library of Congress Cataloging-in-Publication Data

Therapeutic interventions for the person with dementia.

"Has also been published as Physical & occupational therapy in geriatrics, volume 4, no. 3, spring 1986"—T.p. verso.
Includes bibliographies.
1. Alzheimer's disease—Treatment. 2. Senile dementia—Treatment. I. Taira, Ellen. [DNLM: 1. Dementia—therapy. W1 PH683M v.4 no.3 / WM 220 T398]
RC523.T57 1986   618.97'683   86-3123
ISBN 0-86656-556-6

Therapeutic Interventions for the Person with Dementia

Physical & Occupational Therapy in Geriatrics
Volume 4, Number 3

CONTENTS

BOOK REVIEW

FROM THE EDITOR

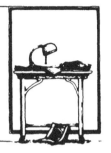

This issue of *POTG* is the realization of a personal and professional goal to reject the "therapeutic nihilism" (Mace) that prevails when rehabilitative intervention is suggested for the demented person.

Therapists specializing in geriatrics have always included the person with senile dementia in restorative treatment programs despite their chronic illness. Failure to respond rarely made the mentally impaired candidates for skilled care yet they often could be maintained at a higher level of functioning with attention to their mobility, self-care and activity needs. The writers for this issue describe approaches to the demented person that reflect a bias towards the rehabilitation of the mentally impaired geriatric patient, regardless of the long term prognosis for their condition.

An advocate of therapeutic intervention for the Alzheimer's victim, Mace gives us a nice overview of the range of possibilities available in the community. This article sets the tone for the rest of the issue which includes some examples of innovative community programming. Rabinowitz's weekend day activity program and Kelley's out patient interdisciplinary team at the Veterans Administration both illustrate a creative approach to non-institutional programs.

Davis' article on the role of therapists with the victim of Alzheimer's disease describes the etiology of the disease, some clinical features of dementia and gives a comprehensive

1

presentation of effective interventions that have proven successful in treatment.

Maloney and Daily's work with a severely impaired group of nursing home residents will be of interest to the new therapist as well as the experienced practitioner with research interests. In contrast to their group work is the article by Griffin and Matthews which focuses on individualizing activities for residents of long term care facilities with special attention to the role of the nurse as an adjunct to therapeutic activities.

The need for environmental modifications is stressed in several of the articles and very thoroughly discussed in the description of the special approach on Wesley Hall by Coons and Weaverdyck. Lastly, Barrett gives a comprehensive discussion of brain-behavior relationships in dementia and the use of the Luria Nebraska Neuropsychological battery as an evaluation, treatment and educational tool.

Some of these approaches are uncharted territory for therapists, yet it is and should be a domain of concern for all rehabilitative professionals interested in geriatrics. As the size of this target group expands and the need to find solutions to their long term care becomes even more pressing than it is now there will be many opportunities for therapeutic intervention. This volume is a first attempt to address the therapeutic needs of the dementia victim. Your comments, criticism and suggestions are welcome.

E. D. T.

Preface

Joan C. Rogers, PhD, OTR

Recently, I was prodded to re-examine my concept of rehabilitation by an article, in a professional publication, which indicated that the biological nature and progressively debilitating course of Alzheimer's Disease precluded rehabilitation. Unfortunately, this attitude can be readily interpreted as suggesting that rehabilitative services are not needed or are inappropriate for this diagnosis. Although cure or even retarding cognitive decline is not presently feasible, the application of rehabilitation philosophy and techniques to patients with Alzheimer's Disease can do much to improve the quality of life of these individuals and of their caregivers.

By assessing the patient's *actual ability* to continue to carry out personal self care and home management tasks, rehabilitation professionals can provide information that is critical for making appropriate decisions regarding independent living, supportive services (i.e., chore workers, meals-on-wheels etc.) guardianship, and least restrictive living situation. In the early stages of Alzheimer's Disease, activities of daily living can often be simplified so that task requirements remain within the person's cognitive capacity to understand them. This simplification may enable the person to use his or her remaining abilities to better advantage to maintain daily living skills. Environmental adaptations can be introduced to make the living situation safe, uncluttered and predictable, and able to serve as a memory aid. When tasks are understood and routinized, stimulus overload can be avoided, and the chances of precipitating catastrophic reactions reduced. If musculoskeletal integrity becomes prob-

Joan C. Rogers, Associate Professor of Occupational Therapy and Assistant Professor of Psychiatry at the Geriatric Psychiatry and Behavioral Neurology Module, Western Psychiatric Institute and Clinic, University of Pittsburgh, Pittsburgh, PA.

lematic, exercise can be prescribed to ward off the deleterious effects of inactivity and make physical care easier. Teaching rehabilitative techniques, such as moving body parts, lifting, and feeding, to caregivers can prevent them from doing harm to the patient or to themselves.

The above examples are a few illustrations of the potential application of rehabilitation to the care and management of patients with Alzheimer's Disease. While they are not consonant with a definition of rehabilitation as a return to former social role functioning, they are in agreement with a conceptualization of rehabilitation as a facilitative process enabling a person with an impairment to remain as independent as possible for as long as possible.

Rehabilitation can project a crucial adjunct to existing intervention for lessening caregiver stress. Rehabilitation can supplement programs designed to improve disease knowledge and can facilitate the expression of feelings and frustrations for those providing training in caregiving skills. This issue of *POTG* offers a variety of treatment interventions for the person with dementia as well as timely and useful information that is easily adaptable to the clinical setting. *Therapeutic Interventions for the Person with Dementia* is a beginning attempt to tap the resources and skills of rehabilitative professionals and apply them to the person with Alzheimer's disease and other related dementias.

Home and Community Services for Alzheimer's Disease

Nancy Mace, MA

It is a personal pleasure to take part in this conference which marks a milestone in our efforts to develop resources for the victims of Alzheimer's disease and their families.

Secretary Heckler has emphasized the need to alleviate the unnecessary disability that poor care and lack of resources inflicts on victims of these diseases. Moreover, she has called for the collaboration of public agencies and families in the war on Alzheimer's disease.

The research into the causes of dementia holds great promise. The improvements in diagnosis and treatment holds immediate promise.

Nevertheless, in the community, families, physicians, nurses and all those who are involved in the care of these patients, still must provide day to day care for the 2–4 million people who are suffering from a uniquely terrible, disabling long term disease.

Federal recognition of the urgency of this problem has doubled the research budget although it remains small in proportion to the care budget. We are spending an estimated 20 billion dollars on nursing home care of dementia victims and an estimated 50 million on basic research into the causes. We are spending even less on research into effective ways to care for patients.

Nancy Mace, MA, Consultant in Gerontology to the Office of Technology Assessment, United States Congress. Co-author, The 36-Hour Day: A Family Guide to Caring for Persons with Alzheimer's Disease, Related Dementing Illnesses and Memory Loss in Later Life.

Reprinted from a speech given at the Alzheimer's Disease and Related Disorders Association National Conference for Families, May 2, 1985, at the National Institutes of Health, Bethesda, MD. Copyrighted by the Alzheimer's Disease and Related Disorders Association.

Despite the increased investment in research, if we do not find a cure or prevention quickly, we will need skills in caring for those who suffer from this devastating illness. We will need to know how best to care for these patients, and how to deliver services to them effectively and equitably, in ways that support the care their families give. Yet, the present system of care delivery often seems to be more afflicted by plaques and tangles than are the brains of those it seeks to serve.

Should we invest our limited resources in research on patient care? Perhaps research into ways to best care for these patients is futile. Perhaps we are already doing as well as can be hoped for in patient care.

Despite the promise offered by the new research in diagnosis, treatment, and cause, one still encounters this attitude of therapeutic nihilism; this feeling that there is nothing we can really do for these patients. We still find those who believe there is nothing to do for those who pace, who scream, who strike out, who weep, except to pour into them chemical straight jackets and wait out the inexorable course of the disease.

This is not true: there is much we can do now, today, to improve the quality of life for these persons—before the discovery of a drug that will slow or reverse the course of the disease.

I watched an interview with a man who was a retired scientist who had early Alzheimer's disease. He was clearly impaired, yet still able to talk about having this illness. He spoke of how he spent his days and he said, "life is good."

Another patient, was maintained at home at considerable cost to his wife and with the coordinated efforts of a medical team and a home health aide. I have a photograph of him sitting with his granddaughter. He did not remember her name, but at that moment he was enjoying that little girl and she was enjoying him.

At a model special unit for victims of dementing illnesses established by Dorothy Coons and her associates, patients showed a decided reduction in incontinence.

> there has been a decided reduction in incontinence by the fifth month most of the persons were sleeping through the night, patients have resumed old household

tasks, become friendly and warm, wandering has been reduced . . . (Coons)

In a survey of day care programs which I conducted at Johns Hopkins, and which was funded by the Wood Kalb foundation, we found that 84% of centers reported that their demented clients made friends at the center; 67% reported that wandering declined; and 71% reported that agitation decreased.

A nursing home administrator who was discussing his special unit for Alzheimer's disease patients, said, "We use fewer medications, and no restraints. The patients are walking and talking and seem much more like their old selves. They make friends and really do very well socially."

Other settings report that some of their patients are remaining mobile until close to the terminal phase of their illness. They report that these patients need fewer psychoactive drugs, catheters and diapers and are less agitated and combative.

Clearly, for some patients, some of the time, having a dementia is not synonymous with suffering. We CAN make a difference in whether such people suffer with their illness or whether they are comfortable and able to enjoy moment to moment.

These success stories are rare. They are far outnumbered by stories of patient and family suffering. I believe that our charge for the coming decade is to learn what we can do to rehabilitate patients, to enable them to live WITH their illness, to improve their function, to remove excess disability, and to improve their quality of life.

We have been saying that home and community programs—day care, board and care, recreation programs in nursing homes, home help, good medical care in hospitals and the approach of the outpatient physician are needed to help keep the patient in situations where his care costs are lower and where families manage without burning out. Now it is time to go further: the best of these programs are THERA-PEUTIC for the patient.

We cannot cure his disease yet, but we cannot cure many diseases. When we cannot cure a chronic disease, we seek to make the patient as functional, as independent, and as comfortable as we can. We teach people with diabetes to change their diet in order to minimize the impact of their disease; we treat depression experienced by a cancer patient and we make the environment accessible to the paraplegic.

To talk about changing the quality of life for the patient as he lives through his illness, we must address two separate issues: (1) what are the techniques of patient care and treatment, and (2) how do we deliver them?

PROVIDING ONGOING CARE AND TREATMENT

First, good patient care and treatment requires a complete and thorough assessment. A complete assessment implies that one thinks one will find some things he can treat. When we fail to assess a patient, we are practicing therapeutic nihilism: we are assuming that there is nothing we can do anyway.

Common sense dictates that any person who is sick should be thoroughly assessed. But too often a person who carries a label of Alzheimer's disease does not receive a thorough assessment. Moreover, when the patient develops other symptoms or illnesses, the worsened condition is blamed on the dementia without enough attention given to the concurrent problems.

Alzheimer's disease is not a new synonym for hopelessness: assessments do identify interventions. Assessment identifies the individual's limitations and it also identifies his strengths and remaining skills. Assessment is an ongoing process. As the patient changes, we must reassess his status, re-identify his areas of spared and impaired function, and repeat the search for concurrent illness.

Second, treat all concurrent illnesses. Persons suffering from dementia need good ongoing medical care. We know that if we keep these patients as well as possible, we enable them to function at their best. For these vulnerable persons, their thinking often worsens when they suffer even minor concurrent illnesses. We must use as few medications as possible, as sparingly as possible, recognizing the risk that medication may further impair function. Successful home and community care depends on the capacity of community physicians to maximize their patients' general health.

Third: treat the patient's disabling symptoms. Patient depression, hallucinations, extreme suspicions, agitation, and wakefulness at night often do respond to treatment interventions.

ENVIRONMENTAL MODIFICATIONS

Fourth: make the patient's environment work for him. Dorothy Coons at the University of Michigan says,

> each of the environmental components—the programs of activities which makes up the daily life of the individual the staff, the physical setting, and other residents—has the potential for becoming a therapeutic or non therapeutic agent in treatment.

A supportive environment recognizes the patients' limited ability to tolerate stress and helps the patient withdraw when demands, noise or confusion become too much for him. A supportive environment reacts with calm and reassurance to disturbed behaviors, it recognizes the patient's need for a social life and offers him ways to maximize old skills.

It may be, as some have theorized, that a barren environment encourages restlessness, agitated, repetitive or socially unacceptable behavior. Furthermore, it appears that, because these patients have limited ability to initiate, organize and plan, they need extensive input from their psychosocial environment to enable them to socialize or do meaningful tasks.

The environment allows for individual choice without too much pressure for difficult decisions; it fills in when a person falters; it simplifies tasks and at the same time provides an opportunity to do meaningful tasks that support a sense of self-worth.

How much more can the environment do? Which physical settings, and which activities support function? What can architects, engineers, product designers and others offer us to help these patients? Can walkers, hearing aids, corrective lenses and incontinence wear be made easier for confused people to use?

To provide a supportive environment for the patient often means helping the caregiver help the patient. An exhausted, stressed caregiver suffers, and so does the patient. Care for the caregiver helps both caregiver and patient.

A number of studies have documented the pressures and burdens that caregivers experience. Women give up jobs to care for their elderly patients; caregivers become exhausted and ill. They may be impoverished and isolated. We know little about the effect of a dementing illness on children in the home, except what one father said of his children, "It sure didn't help them."

Recently, a caregiving wife called me. She was 72, and had been caring for her husband for ten years. He had suddenly developed fecal incontinence, become combative, and was often awake and agitated most of the night. She had finally decided to seek nursing home placement, only to discover she would be required to impoverish herself to pay for his care.

The real tragedy is he was probably suffering from an acute illness which had exacerbated his systems. Had I been able to refer her to a dementia treatment team these people could have been helped. Good care requires special skills and, so far, is extremely rare. The first step in rehabilitation is often to advocate for making patients as physically well as possible.

CONTINUUM OF CARE

We need a continuum of care resource. We have models for these services but they are too few to serve the estimated two million patients and their families.

We need good medical care in the emergency room, the acute hospital, and in out patient settings. Studies have revealed that dementia is not noticed by clinicians in the emergency room and is not always diagnosed in in patient acute settings. How can we treat the patient if we don't notice that his thinking is impaired?

Most Alzheimer's disease victims live at home. We need help at home. This may include visiting multidisciplinary teams; it may include trained people who can take the patient for walks, play tennis with him, or just sit with him while the family member gets out. Such in home care can be more than a sitter service; it can be an opportunity to initiate therapeutic interventions that the exhausted caregiver cannot provide.

We need short term respite care—someone who can stay overnight for several days in the home, while the family caregiver is away. We need more day care: where the patient can socialize, where he senses that he is both accepted and is making a contribution—a place that relieves the caregiving family for a few hours, a place where the impaired person can make friends.

We need residential board and care—where the patient can live in a setting that makes him feel at home, allows him to feel useful and secure, where setting the table is still something she can do—a place that does not demand intellectual skills but supports social skills. It may be a residential setting that provides medical and nursing care as well as structure, safety, comfort and peace with carefully supervised medication, no restraints, good diet and good skin care.

We need hospice programs where one's final weeks are supported with compassion and understanding.

We need police and ambulance crews who know how to help when they are called upon in emergencies. We need nursing home aides who understand what life is like for a victim of Alzheimer's disease.

Community and home care include the provision of legal protection for the patient. When he can no longer take responsibility for himself, he must have legal and financial help that takes into consideration his humanity, his freedom, his dignity and his needs.

THERAPEUTIC INTERVENTION

Others have pointed out that we have only just begun to explore the potential of rehabilitation: speech therapy, physical therapy, occupational therapy and other therapies in helping patients compensate for their disability. Rehabilitation for these patients is different from rehabilitation of a person fully able to learn new skills. We need therapists with the talent to search out new ways to help memory impaired people.

High tech may also offer resources to help our patients. Certainly we don't want to replace tender loving care with robots but we have not yet begun to explore what these technologies can offer our patients. Just improvements in the technology of managing incontinence would be welcomed by caregivers.

We need policies which support service delivery research and innovative experimental patient care techniques. We need to analyze what the good programs do and how they do it. We need to know how much care costs, what the limitations of each kind of care are—patient tolerance and fatigue, long distances to transport patients, family exhaustion and stress.

INFORMATION DISSEMINATION

We need policies which encourage the dissemination of information. We need to spread this knowledge widely and quickly and to systematically share what we learn, rapidly, generously and efficiently. We need to develop a large cadre of people trained in the new skills as fast as the new skills are developed.

It is unlikely that we can do this with a fragmented, 19th century system of communicating. Other disciplines have discovered the value of computer communications in settings where rapid change in the knowledge base occurs. A system somewhat like a computer bulletin board used by researchers and care providers would be a relatively cost effective and fast way to exchange information about techniques, deliver current information to new programs and broaden the base of patients from which we can learn.

We need policy which guarantees that services are coordinated. Fragmented unnetworks will not help us care for these patients. There are too many difficulties in their care, it is too costly and too overwhelming a problem to risk the kind of fragmentation and competition that has marred other public programs.

QUALITY ASSURANCE

We need to address the difficult issues of quality assurance. Alzheimer's disease is a big name now—that is good—and we hope for funds to create new programs. We need to begin now to think about ways to ensure that the new, experimental, caring programs have the flexibility to try innovative techniques but at the same time guarantee quality. At present we do not have uniformly adequate standards for patient safety in case of fire, and humane patient care. In some states there are no standards at all for some kinds of respite services.

We must ensure safety, good health, and hopefully good programs. To design quality assurance policies that will ensure quality care will challenge the best minds but professionals and families must start now to demand it.

The recognition that there are things we can do now to improve the quality of life for victims of a dementing illness makes it absolutely essential that we have policy which ensures equality of access to services. Across the nation I have heard families say that access to services is not equitable: that the cost of services bankrupts them; that the tasks of caring exhausts them emotionally and physically.

These ideas will require major changes in our mindset and an even greater change in our fiscal policy. We have no grounds to take a stance of therapeutic nihilism because we do not have a cure for Alzheimer's or for multi-infarct dementia.

There is much that we can do to treat and care for victims of dementing illness. There are excellent treatment teams, legal talent, day care centers, respite programs, residential settings, Alzheimer units. There is much we have only begun to think of—the tools of high tech and of rehabilitation medicine.

REFERENCES

Coons, D. H. et al., The Family Connection: A Handbook for Family Visiting, in press.

Mace, N. and Rabins, P. "A Survey of Day Care for the Demented Adult in the United States," National Council on Aging, Washington, D.C., 1984.

Coons, D. "Milieu Therapy, The Social Psychological Aspects of Treatment" in Reichel, W. The Clinical Aspects of Aging, 1978, Baltimore: Williams and Wilkins.

The Role of the Physical and Occupational Therapist in Caring for the Victim of Alzheimer's Disease

Carol M. Davis, EdD, PT

ABSTRACT. The threats that dementia present to us as caregivers center mainly on the lack of predictability of the client's day-to-day responses and the overwhelming sense of loss of a meaningful life as victims regress before our eyes without any sense of hope for cure. The goals of our care must be focused on maintaining as high a quality of life as possible for as long as possible. Interventions are outlined and suggestions are made to help communicate through catastrophic reactions, depression and confusion. The methods of validation therapy are suggested to be superior to reality therapy in communicating acceptance and support for the demented patient who will never again know reality as we know it.

What is it about dementia that seems to threaten us, especially those of us who have not been trained in psychiatry? Few who care for confused demented elderly clients deny a feeling of anxiety and dread, sometimes pity that seems not to be present in caring for those with other physical illnesses. Some might say their anxiety stems from a lack of predictability in the client's behavior, others speak of a feeling of helplessness in breaking through the fog of confusion. Many of us would "choose" more physically debilitating aging processes over "losing our minds." At the core of the frustration that we feel is undoubtedly the reality that, as we care for these

---

Carol M. Davis, Assistant Professor, Acting Co-chair, Department of Physical Therapy, Sargent College, Boston University, One University Road, Boston, MA 02215.

people, we are forced to stand by and watch the life of a person disintegrate before our very eyes.

> Personhood, of necessity, requires intact cortical structure. . . . [B]iological life prolongation becomes of secondary importance since it is only organic life that is here prolonged, not the life of a person. (Spicker, 1978)

Unlike most other syndromes we involve ourselves with, organic brain disease, including Alzheimer's, offers no semblance of hope for recovery.

As occupational and physical therapists, the meaning in our work takes life in our connectedness with persons, not with bodies. How can we prepare ourselves to be therapeutically present for victims of dementia in spite of their predictable downhill course? This article is written with the belief that the more we can predict what to expect from these patients, and the more clearly we understand appropriate responses to their unpredictable behavior, the more adequate can our therapeutic responses be. The goal, at all times, is to maintain the quality of their lives at the highest level possible for the duration of their decline.

In this paper I will briefly review the epidemiology and histopathology associated with Alzheimer's disease and the three hypotheses often thought to be associated with the etiology. I will also review the clinical features differentiating pseudodementia from dementia. But the focus of this paper is intended to be on the predictable progression of symptoms, and the interactive interventions that have been shown to be effective, including the particular forms and styles of communication that can "break through" the fog of confusion and depression.

EPIDEMIOLOGY

According to Glenner, organic brain syndrome, with its symptoms of confusion, decline in memory, disorientation, confabulation, and depression, affects over 1.5 million American adults at an estimated cost of 20 billion dollars each year. Sixty percent of all cases of dementia are due to Alzheimer's disease, seventeen percent are due to multi-infarct phenomena along with Alzheimer's and ten percent of all cases of dementia are due to multi-infarct disease alone. "One family in every three will see one of their parents succumb to this disease" (Glenner, 1982). Alzheimer's disease is the fourth most common cause of death in the United States. The symptoms are insidiously slow and can progress over a period of four to fifteen years with a mean of 8 years. Only the very wealthy or the very poor escape being financially broken from the overwhelming cost of maintaining the quality of life during this period of decline.

DIAGNOSIS AND ETIOLOGY

Symptoms of Alzheimer's disease start with loss of recent memory or distortion of memory of recent events. Disorientation, first to time and place, then to person, follows along with loss of more remote memory with the victim exhibiting denial and attempting to cover up the problem as part of the fear of "losing one's mind." Eventually only the memory of pain is preserved as all loss of sensation and kinesthetic sense becomes involved (Glenner, 1982). Table 1 reviews the progression of symptoms over a period of time from diagnosis to a complete vegetative state often setting the stage for death from pneumonia.

The elderly often show signs of depression, endogenous and/or situational, either as result of dealing with multiple losses and/or as a side effect to various medications. Depression can cause a blunting of affect and a diminishing of the amount of energy one wants to give to day to day living. This depressed state often masks as a dementia, or can be regarded as a pseudodementia, and can be mistaken for the true dementia of Alzheimer's disease. Table 2 summarizes the critical differences between these two syndromes.

Conclusive diagnosis of Alzheimer's disease can be made only by biopsy or autopsy. Gross examination of brain tissue reveals cortical atrophy and dilated ventricles with altered dendritic morphology (loss of dendritic spines, dying of dendrites and swelling of neuronal somata), granulovacuolar degeneration (mainly in hippocampal pyramidal cells and in the

Dementia: The loss of ability to be responsive for directing one's daily life.
Delirium: Rather abrupt changes in mental state, fluctuating alertness, confusion.

Forgetful	Confused	Vegetative
X		

| Symptoms: | Diagnosis | 4-15 years ($\overline{X}$=8 yrs) |

Impairment of recent memory------increases-----------------------

Disorientation to time and place---------and person-----------

Retrogressive loss of remote memory-----------------------

apraxia/anomia/aphasia/agnosia

Confabulation relevant to habitual premorbid activity---

All sensory and kinesthetic function becomes involved
except the memory of pain

Driving becomes difficult and then impossible

"Getting lost"----------------apraxia with use of car, keys

Reasoning deteriorates---depression, agitation-------
irritability, restlessness

Degeneration in concentration, speech, walking----
hand writing

Violence----placid, inertia

Disruption in sleep/awake cycles----------------

Total inability to care for self
incontinence, pneumonia, urinary
tract infection, death

Table 1.   Progression of symptoms over a period of four
to fifteen years with Alzheimer's disease

medial temporal gyri) and neuritic or senile plaques (microscopic, spherical accumulation of cellular and extracellular debris) (DeBoni and McLachlan, 1980).

In addition gray matter cells of the cortex display within them paired helical filaments (PHF's) or tangles. The greater the number of tangles and plaques, the more severe is the extent of intellectual impairment (Glenner, 1982).

The etiology of these brain cell changes is unknown. No animal model is known to exist. Glenner notes that progress in discovering a cause and/or cure to Alzheimer's disease is thwarted by the tendency to attribute the symptoms to normal aging processes and/or cerebral arteriosclerosis. Neither, of course, is the case. Obtaining biopsy specimens is difficult because patients often have deteriorated to the extent that they cannot give legal consent (Glenner, 1982).

Three hypotheses regarding etiology identified by DeBoni and associates include: (1) a pathologic event which reduces

TABLE 2 CLINICAL FEATURES DIFFERENTIATING
PSEUDODEMENTIA FROM DEMENTIA*

Pseudodementia	Dementia
Clinical Course and History	
1. Family always aware of dysfunction and its severity	1. Family often unaware of dysfunction and its severity
2. Onset can be dated with some precision	2. Onset can be dated only within broad limits
3. Symptoms of short duration before medical help is sought	3. Symptoms usually of long duration before medical help is sought
4. Rapid progression of symptoms after onset	4. Slow progression of symptoms throughout course
5. History of previous psychiatric dysfunction common	5. History of previous psychiatric dysfunction unusual
Complaints and Clinical Behavior	
1. Patients usually complain much of cognitive loss	1. Patients usually complain little of cognitive loss
2. Patients complaints of cognitive dysfunction usually detailed	2. Patients complaints of cognitive dysfunction usually vague
3. Patients emphasize disability	3. Patients conceal disability
4. Patients highlight gailures	4. Patients delight in accomplishments, however trivial
5. Patients make little effort to perform even simple tasks	5. Patients struggle to perform tasks
6. Patients don't try to keep up	6. Patients rely on notes, calendars, etc., to keep up
7. Patients usually communicate strong sense of distress	7. Patients often appear unconcerned
8. Affective change often pervasive	8. Affect labile and shallow
9. Loss of social skills often early and prominent	9. Social skills often retained
10. Behavior often incongruent with severity of cognitive dysfunction	10. Behavior usually compatible with severity of cognitive dysfunction
11. Nocturnal accentuation of dysfunction uncommon	11. Nocturnal accentuation of dysfunction common
Clinical Features Related to Memory, Cognitive and Intellectual Dysfunctions	
1. Attention and concentration often well preserved	1. Attention and concentration usually faulty
2. "Don't know" answers typical	2. "Near miss" answer frequent
3. On tests of orientation, patients often give "don't know" answers	3. On tests of orientation, patients often mistake unusual for usual
4. Memory loss for recent and remote events usually equally severe	4. Memory loss for recent events usually more severe than for remote events
5. Memory gaps for specific periods or events common	5. Memory gaps for specific periods unusual
6. Marked variability in performance on tasks of similar difficulty	6. Consistently poor performance on tasks of similar difficulty

*From Wells, C.E.: The differential diagnosis of psychiatric disorders in the elderly. In Cole, J.O. and Barrett, J.E. (eds): Psychopathology of the aged. New York, Raven Press, 1980, with permission.

the amount of RNA produced by the cell nucleus, (2) "a primary event resulting in the assembly of paired helical filaments (PHF's) with a concomitant reduction in the number of microtubules and secondarily resulting in a reduction of dendroplasmic transport, and (3) a defect in the blood barrier permitting the accumulation within brain parenchyma of potentially toxic environmental compounds, including trace metals" (DeBoni, 1980). Each of these possible causes may be associated with viral infection. Direct injection of diseased tissue into unaffected animals has yet to produce the disease. Larger than usual amounts of the toxic substance aluminum has been discovered in Alzheimer's brain tissue but research shows that although aluminum causes brain atrophy, it does not induce PHF's nor neuritic plaques (DeBoni, 1980). Genetic studies reveal that "family numbers of an Alzheimer's disease patient have a 4.3 times greater chance of getting the disease than does the general population" (Glenner, 1982).

The end result of the pathological changes in the brain cells of Alzheimer's victims is a reduction of choline acetyltransferase which converts choline into acetylcholine, necessary for memory. Treatment by injection of this enzyme into brain tissue is prevented by the tremendous instability of the substance. Thus attempts are currently being undertaken to give oral doses of physostigmine which prevents the breakdown of acetylcholine. This research is showing slightly optimistic results (Sevush, in press).

GOALS OF CARE

How do we, as occupational and physical therapists, make a difference in the care of our clients with Alzheimer's disease? At the outset we must be committed to a thorough evaluation of each client to obtain a complete and individual sense of their existing deficit. Each client is uniquely different, and until we understand the complete nature of his or her deficit, we cannot undertake a meaningful plan of care. Physical symptoms will likely be minimal at first. A mental status examination is central to the evaluation process (Folstein, 1975).

The world is full of potential hazards for Alzheimer's victims. An evaluation of the client's living environment and a thorough Activities of Daily Living evaluation will offer clues to problems with function that the client's family needs to be made aware of. Key questions that should be addressed might include:

—Might the client mistake hot for cold water?
—Can he or she answer the phone or doorbell?
—What self care problems are likely?

> Dressing, grooming?
> Handling zippers, buttons?
> Finding clothes to put on; putting them on in proper sequence?
> Use of washcloth, soap, toothbrush, comb?

—Can the client handle stairs?
—What about walking outside?

> Will he/she get lost?
> Can he/she handle shopping?
> Make change?
> Understand a list?

—Can the client tell time? Understand time passage?
—What about safety?

> Gates, locks, rails necessary?

—Should knives or sharp objects be removed?

Attention must be focused on a thorough evaluation of the client's sensory deficit. What is the nature of the sensory loss, if any? Can the client see, with or without glasses? Or is the problem that he or she can see, but not interpret what is seen? The same is true for hearing, touch, taste and smell.

An adjunct to the retrogressive loss of memory is the development of the four "a" symptoms: agnosia, anomia, apraxia and aphasia. *Agnosia* is the loss of comprehension of sensation even though the sensory apparatus remains intact. Clients cannot interpret sounds, images seen or objects touched or smelled. Most poignant is the inability to recognize what should be familiar faces, names or events. *Anomia* is the inability to remember names and the misuse of names or words. *Apraxia* is the inability to perform learned motor acts or the "out of the ordinary" actions that surprise us and seem inappropriate. *Aphasia* is the inability to express oneself appropriately, often not a disruption in speech as is common with cerebrovascular accident, but a loss of memory for words or an inability to articulate certain words or an utterance of meaningless phrases or gibberish. Often clients know what they want to say but can't say it. In the early stages they may exhibit frustration or try to hide these symptoms. As the disease progresses, the frustration may lead to violent outbursts and then to a placid inertia and apathy.

"Environmental press" is a phenomenon that demands attention with Alzheimer's victims. Caretakers must be helped to understand that sensory overload or an increase in the number and complexity of demands on Alzheimer's victims will frustrate them. This may take place with more than one person in the room speaking or moving, with a three or four step request of the client or with voices, music and other noises stressing the client all at one time. When this occurs the environment must be modified to decrease the sensory demand. This problem is discussed in more detail later.

HELPING CLIENTS LEARN

Alzheimer's victims are capable of learning in spite of their deficits. The keys to teaching them include the use of one stage requests followed by appropriate pauses to let the request register. Memory cues and sensory adjuncts are very helpful. Labels on drawers, doors, by the telephone help keep the confusing world more manageable. It often takes up to two weeks for them to learn a new skill. Praise and encouragement are critical to learning; we must never use criticism or negative reinforcement. "You're doing it all wrong" has no meaning to one who has no idea what right or wrong is. Consistency is critical. If we want the client to use a cane or walker, we must request that he or she use it 100 percent of the time. As we instruct the family we must ask them to gently assist, to fill in the gaps without resentment. Choosing to believe the client is doing the best he or she can at the moment is imperative. We must learn to work with Alzheimer's victims as we would with a child and yet honor him or her as an adult. The more a client's children need him or her to be their parent, the more difficult this new way of relating will be. Family members should also be reinforced, supported and praised for their efforts.

HANDLING CATASTROPHIC REACTIONS

A common response to stress of Alzheimer's clients is a catastrophic reaction or a refusal to cooperate, often accompanied by screams, crying, violent outbursts of anger with attempts to strike out or throw things. The etiology of the catastrophic reaction is sensory or cognitive overload, misinterpretation of sensory information or a request, and fatigue or frustration with the inability to perform a task. The client cannot change; we must act to reduce the reaction. Getting the client's attention by verbalizing what's happening right now with the assurance, "You are safe, you are all right," is a good place to start. Information must be given clearly, slowly and simply, one step at a time. Stand where the client can see you; never approach from behind. Reduce noise or activity, reduce the number of choices the client must make, limit the amount or number of items of food on the client's plate or on the table. Restructure the environment to reduce stress. Avoid arguing, respond sympathetically to his or her stress. If the client has picked an object up and is about to throw it, clap your hands and state sharply, "Look! Behind you!" Often they will forget they were about to be violent and will calm down. If environmental modifications cease to reduce the reaction, it's time to consider medication. Reinforce to the family that the client is *not* in control of his or her behavior and they are not to personalize these outbursts.

MANAGING SUSPICIOUSNESS

Alzheimer's victims struggle moment to moment to make sense out of a very confusing world. They tend to misinterpret ordinary activities as an attack on them, as sexual behavior, or as a theft of their possessions. This leads to bizarre responses and uncooperativeness as we try to care for them. Often they harbor fixed delusions that are tenacious and resist logic or explanation. To argue may exacerbate a catastrophic reaction. Take time to establish rapport and trust. This is the only factor that will influence them. Reassure the family, again, that they are not responsive to reason. Trust is a complex human emotion that requires memory to be sustained. Patience and gentle reassurance in the moment is the most we can offer. Medication once again must be considered.

UNDERSTANDING APATHY

Eventually Alzheimer's victims slip into an inert apathetic existence. They may resist getting out of bed or partaking in activity as they once did. This may be due to a fear of falling, fear of the confusing world, or it may also be due to further brain deterioration, depression or delirium. In the final stages of the disease clients are totally unable to care for themselves and become lethargic and incontinent. But before this total degeneration takes hold, apathy may be reversed by a careful examination for depression secondary to the side effects of medication or response to loss. The quality of the day to day life of the client demands that apathy be understood and reversed if at all possible.

COMMUNICATING WITH THE CLIENT WITH ALZHEIMER'S DISEASE

Remember that apraxia is the inability to complete a motor task. To assist the client, break down the task into its simplest parts and gently communicate what to do in one stage commands.

With agnosia, communicating information in gentle and undemanding ways may help the client feel more at ease with his or her memory loss. Not reacting negatively when a person is not recognized is difficult but important in sustaining the client's self esteem. Friends and family members need support as they experience a lifetime of loving memories fade away from the person they've shared so much with.

In the presence of aphasia, filling in the missing word may help decrease tension and frustration. Family and other caretakers must learn the meaning of each client's idiosyncratic phrases. "I want to go home" may mean, "I don't know where I am." Responding with "But you *are* home" may not be as helpful as, "I can tell you're anxious about where you are right now. You are safe. This is our living room and you belong here with us."

Watch the client for signs of anxiety or pain. Ask if he or she has pain and wait for a response before you ask, "Where?" If the person says, "No" but you suspect may mean yes, ask the person to point to where it hurts to see if they may be miscommunicating with their words. Demonstrate what you want them to do.

Again, sensory and memory problems can best be communicated through using simple one step commands or one stage instructions, several sensory cues, giving the client plenty of time to respond.

COMMUNICATING WITH THE DEPRESSED CLIENT

Symptoms of depression may include a loss of interest in one's surroundings, lack of initiative, preoccupation with one's physical or physiological state and/or loneliness, lack of purpose or meaning.

Maizler suggests that, as care givers, our principle role with depressed patients, confused or not, is to listen with undivided attention conveying the attitude that, "You are important to me." In brief he suggests:

1. Be clear about time. Convey exactly how much time you can spend with them.
2. Allow expression of feeling.
3. Communicate your understanding that sometimes we can't help feeling this way.
4. Reinforce dignity. Accept anger without reaction.
5. Be congruent with your verbal and nonverbal messages and feelings. If you don't have the time or can't give the attention fully, don't try to give half heartedly.
6. Use touch to convey support, caring (Maizler, 1982).

With older people we may find ourselves needing our clients to act in ways we unconsciously expect from our parents. Likewise, children of Alzheimer's victims have a great task to achieve in overcoming their need to be parented by people who, for all intents, are no longer able to parent anyone.

COMMUNICATING THROUGH CONFUSION

The confused demented client is often rendered more frustrated by our attempts to confront him or her with reality. These people need not be made to realize that this is 1985 in order to regain an ability to function adequately in the world of today. The fact is they are only going to become more confused and our assaults on them with reality do little to help them and usually represent a need to reduce *our* anxiety. Naomi Feil recounts this dialogue as a good example:

> Mr. K: Hey John, fix the basement steps. Your mom just tripped and hurt her knee.
>
> Physician: I'm not your son John, Mr. K., I'm the doctor who is examining you.
>
> Mr. K: Oh shut up you bastard and fix the steps.

Feil offers: "Confronting the patient with present reality is unhelpful. The disoriented person in this instance has decided to retreat because he cannot bear the many losses that accumulate with age." She suggests the following as a more appropriate response:

> Mr. K: Hey John, fix the basement steps. Your mother just tripped.
>
> Physician: Did your wife trip, Mr. K? Was she hurt bad? I remind you of your son John. Do I look like him?
>
> Mr. K: Yeah. You're John all right. Boy she never was the same. The old girl just conked right out after that fall (Feil, 1984).

Feil suggests that the client is thus given the chance to express old feelings of guilt after his wife's fall. "The physician is certain of his own reality, and can afford to step into Mr. K's shoes to create a feeling of empathy" (Feil, 1984).

With the client who uses nondictionary words that seem personally constructed Feil suggests "repeating the words, emphasizing the key words in their sentences."

> There are three needs in particular that these patients seem most often to express:
>
> —the need to belong
> —the need to be useful
> —the need to express strong feelings of anger, sadness or love. (Feil, 1984)

She offers this example:

> Mrs. K: This Fendalle company doesn't distangle the messy congruents.
>
> Physician: Mrs. K, does the Fendalle company bother you? Are the congruents too messy?
>
> Mrs. K: Meaningful friends from the company will untangle the mess in the noodles of the brain.
>
> Physician: Do you mean that you miss your company? Is that what Fendalle means?
>
> Mrs. K: Yes, memorable friends from the past.
>
> Physician: We can take a trip to the past using the imagination, can't we?
>
> Mrs. K: Oh yes. And the company will pay the fare. They always do.

For those of us educated from the reality therapy perspective Feil's approach, termed validation therapy, may seem contrary to our training, but in the final analysis it makes more sense. Clients respond to validation therapy with increased attention in the present to the one communicating rather than seeing the communicator as an adversary. The support, understanding and acceptance of validation therapy for those who will never again experience reality as we know it contributes to the quality of their day to day existence in ways reality therapy could never accomplish.

SUMMARY

And what is our task in the face of the inevitable disintegration of a person before our very eyes? To maintain the quality of life, day to day, at the highest level possible. Responding to each person and each family with personal support, advice and attention is the best we can offer victims of Alzheimer's disease. The better we know ourselves and the more genuine and congruent we can be, the better the care we'll be able to give.

REFERENCES

DeBoni, U., McLachlan, D.R.C. Senile dementia and Alzheimer's disease: a current view. *Life Sciences,* 1980, 27, 1–14.

Feil, N. Communicating with the confused elderly patient. *Geriatrics,* 1984, 39, 131–132.

Folstein, M. D., Folstein, S. E., McHugh, P. R. Mini Mental State: a practical method for grading the cognitive state of patients for the clinician. *J. Psychiatric Res.,* 1975, 12, 189–198.

Glenner, G. G. Alzheimer's disease (senile dementia): a research update and critique with recommendations. *Journal of the American Geriatrics Society,* 1982, 30, 59–62.

Maizler, J. S. Mourning and maturity in later life. *Continuing Education,* 1982, April, 23–24.

Sevush S., Morton, C., Guterman, A., Villalone, A. V. Dementia of the Alzheimer's type: improved verbal learning following out patient oral physostigmine therapy. *Neurology,* in press.

Spicker, S. F. Gerontologic mentation: memory, dementia and medicine in the penultimate years. In Spicker, S. F., Wordward, K. M., Van Tassell, D. D., eds. *Aging and the Elderly-Humanistic Perspectives in Gerontology.* Cleveland: Case Western Reserve University, 1978.

Wesley Hall:
A Residential Unit for Persons with Alzheimer's Disease and Related Disorders

Dorothy H. Coons, BS
Shelly E. Weaverdyck, MA

ABSTRACT. Too frequently the impairment of persons with dementia is considered to be caused exclusively by organic brain change. The impact of environmental intervention on functional impairment due to dementia and the need for professionally developed environmental intervention programs are beginning to be recognized.

This paper describes a model residential treatment project for persons with Alzheimer's disease and related dementias designed and implemented by staff of the Institute of Gerontology, the University of Michigan. This research/demonstration project, called Wesley Hall, is structured to maximize capacities, compensate for deficits, and foster success and self-respect on the part of residents. The description of the model identifies interventions or combinations of interventions that have been effective in reducing such behaviors as incontinence, restlessness and anxiety reactions. The project rejects the medical diagnosis of dementia alone as a basis for determining treatment. A case profile of one of the residents illustrates the value of designing individualized milieu intervention programs based on extensive knowledge about each person gained from observation and neuropsychological testing.

Dorothy H. Coons is Project Director, Institute of Gerontology, and Associate Professor Emeritus of Education, the University of Michigan, 300 North Ingalls Building, Ann Arbor, MI 48109-2997; Shelly E. Weaverdyck is Neuropsychology and Research Consultant for the Wesley Hall project at the Institute of Gerontology, the University of Michigan and Ph.D candidate.

Other project staff of the Institute of Gerontology, the University of Michigan, include Anne Robinson, Director of the Wesley Hall Unit, and Beth Spencer, Program Consultant.

29

Much of the literature on dementia in old age focuses on the frailties and deficits of victims, on the loss of cognitive abilities, and on the problem behaviors which accompany the decline in functional capacities. This characterization and treatment of dementia is usually presented in a medical context, which assumes that deficits result from the brain damage and are, thus, inevitable and untreatable. This assumption is now being questioned by a number of American and European researchers. Haugen (1985) of Norway, for example, asks "To what extent is the mental decline a result of passivity, loss of friends, relatives, and spouse? Is the old person able to find support in the resources of the environment? For instance, to what extent does the environment provide stimulation and activation . . .?" Hellebrandt (1978) of the United States believes that "confusion and dependency may be attributable to a combination of isolation, sensory deprivation, immobility, muscle weakness, visual, and auditory deficits."

Wood and Britton (1985) of Great Britain in discussing the impact of stimulating programs on persons with dementia state: "If dementia can be seen as arising from the interaction of impaired recent memory and deprivation of sensory stimulation and environmental input, then increasing the amount of stimulation and activity may be a means of reducing confused behavior."

The study by Brody et al. (1973) suggests the need for environmental therapeutic interventions for persons with dementia. In reporting on their findings and the implications for practitioners they state: "The existence of excess disabilities that are accessible to treatment intervention signifies that the diagnostic label of chronic brain syndrome should indicate treatment intervention, not benign neglect."

Earlier research of the Institute of Gerontology, the University of Michigan, in the use of the therapeutic milieu as a treatment agent with elderly mental hospital patients and later their exploratory studies of persons with dementia (Coons, 1983), suggest that the physical and social environments are significant factors in the care and treatment of elderly dementia victims. These early studies demonstrated the importance of grouping persons with similar needs and capabilities in order to design an environment and way of life that would be therapeutic for them. The studies further suggested the importance of providing the elderly with opportunities to continue in normal social roles even though they might be in need of medical care. The contribution of medical care in a dementia treatment program should be similar to that in society at large; it is essential to optimal physical and mental health but it does not become the primary orientation.

Social roles suggest appropriate behaviors and define society's expectations. If a treatment setting provides only the opportunity for the elderly person to assume the role of "patient," it states clearly that the individual is expected to be sick. On the other hand, if the setting offers a variety of opportunities to continue in normal social roles, for example, friend, homemaker, family member, and volunteer, the expectations are that the older person will continue to function in normal ways to the extent possible and thus deserve the respect attributed to "normal" persons. The implication is that each individual still has a degree of wellness which staff recognize and value.

Wesley Hall, a residential treatment unit for elderly persons with Alzheimer's disease and related dementias, was designed and implemented as a demonstration project by the Institute of Gerontology, as a part of its ongoing investigation of appropriate models for impaired elderly persons. Wesley Hall emphasizes social and physical milieu interventions in its attempt to minimize and compensate for deficits and maximize capacities.

This paper will give a brief description of Wesley Hall and the range of opportunities available to residents living in the area. It will identify the interventions or combinations of interventions that have been effective in reducing the frequency of several selected behaviors considered characteristic of Alzheimer's disease. And finally, a case profile of a resident on Wesley Hall will be presented demonstrating the abilities of persons with dementia to manage a variety of tasks, express emotions and respond in normal ways. The profile also illustrates the project's rejection of a medical diagnosis alone as a basis for determining treatment and demonstrates the value of designing an individualized milieu intervention program based on an extensive body of knowledge about each person gained by observation and neuropsychological testing.

THE DEVELOPMENT OF WESLEY HALL

The idea for Wesley Hall was conceived when it was determined by an administrator of a home for the aged that at least 10 percent of the 150 residents in that home were having such severe memory problems that they were unable to cope in the large, and for them, overwhelming environment in which they were expected to manage with a minimum of staff assistance. Added to their difficulties of orientation were the reactions of well residents who became increasingly angry and frustrated by their constant wandering, bursts of anger and combativeness, and incontinence.

Wesley Hall, opened in December of 1983, is a specially designed residential area for persons with Alzheimer's disease and similar dementias. Housing eleven residents, nine women and two men, it occupies the top (fourth) floor of one wing of a retirement home. This floor of the retirement home was selected because it was separated from the rest of the home and did not serve as a thoroughfare as did other wings. It also had two areas that could be converted to public space, one for a living room with a connected dining room area and a second for a small den. It would have been preferable to have a unit which had direct access to the outdoors, but no such area was available.

Because the retirement home was a very old building with poor lighting, old plumbing and glossy tile floors, Wesley Hall was completely renovated in preparation for the project. Ceilings were lowered and lighting doubled. The living room, den, and dining area were furnished with homelike furniture, and a small kitchen was installed which was to become the hub of much activity. Wallpaper was used in the living room, kitchen, hall, den and bathrooms to provide a warm, non-institutional appearance. Gradually, as needs became apparent, signs were installed to direct residents to specific areas, to call attention to the contributions each resident makes to the daily life, and to help maintain personal identification. A number of photographs made of residents' involvement in the various activities were enlarged and hung to form a gallery in the hall. Residents frequently comment on the pictures. This provides residents and staff with opportunities to reminisce about the good times they have had together.

The Staffing Pattern

The Wesley Hall staff, all employed by the retirement home, were carefully trained by the Institute of Gerontology staff in preparation for the project. Weekly problem-solving sessions have been held to deal with difficult situations that arise. Wesley Hall staff include one full-time and one half-time resident assistant on both the day shift and the evening shift, one resident assistant on the night shift, one full-time coordinator, supportive nursing services for administering medications and monitoring medical problems, and a part-time housekeeper. Most of the resident assistants were selected from the aides employed by the retirement home and its adjacent nursing home area. Their titles were changed from aides to resident assistants to reflect their new non-medical roles.

The physician, who is the medical director of the retirement home, evaluates each resident on Wesley Hall and prescribes medical treatment. He has worked closely with Wesley Hall staff since the beginning of the project. The retirement home, unfortunately, does not employ an occupational or physical therapist.

Selection of Wesley Hall Residents

All staff from the retirement home, housekeeping, dietary, nursing, activities, and administration made recommendations of persons whom they felt could benefit from a residence in the Wesley Hall environment. Project staff interviewed those most frequently mentioned and selected residents to move into the new area. The selection criteria included the following: The resident (a) is ambulatory; (b) is able to feed him/herself; (c) gives evidence of having severe memory loss; (d) does not require more than the minimum amount of medical care that can be administered by the limited number of staff; (e) can manage some self-care with the assistance of staff; (f) can follow instructions related to very simple tasks such as pouring a glass of milk or putting cookies on a plate.

Of the eleven residents originally selected, eight had had a diagnosis of Alzheimer's disease; two multi-infarct dementia; and one, dementia secondary to viral encephalitis.

Early screening procedures were less elaborate than those eventually developed, resulting in the selection of two residents among the first eleven who were far more impaired than the early screening methods revealed. They could not respond to the area, and were in need of far more nursing care than the area could provide with limited staff. The two moved to nursing homes as have others when physical illness increased their need for care. Five of the original eleven still live in the area, and all but one are doing remarkably well. All are needing greater assistance from staff than on first admission in self-care activities and in handling other tasks. Staff believe, however, that verbal skills have improved for many, and they are more responsive and aware of others.

Life on Wesley Hall

It is generally assumed that one of the essentials in providing a therapeutic environment for persons with Alzheimer's disease is the reduction of stress. Mace and Rabins (1981) discuss the need to maintain a calm and relaxed approach in responding to persons with dementia. Loftus (1980), in pointing out that stress hinders accurate perception and memory, states that "Under high stress, people concentrate on fewer features in their environment, and thus many features get less attention. So much energy is expended on anxiety that not much is left over for coping with anything else." The range of opportunities and activities described below, which reinstate normal social roles, might appear overwhelming to residents and therefore stressful. This has not been the case, however. The presence of opportunities has created a therapeutic environment. Conversely, it follows that the absence of such opportunities is non-therapeutic. Institute project staff are convinced that an environment *without* any meaningful activities is stressful and encourages many of the behaviors that are labeled as "problems," "inappropriate," and "sick." Staff use a gentle, encouraging and supportive approach, and coercion or attempts to control residents are considered inappropriate and non-therapeutic.

Wesley Hall was designed to be as non-institutional as possible by creating a home-like physical environment, by promoting individuality, by emphasizing capacities, and by fostering self-respect and as much control on the part of each resident as possible. Stress was reduced by carefully tailoring each activity to what residents could manage successfully and by giving them the option to accept or reject involvement at anytime.

Programming on Wesley Hall

Programming on Wesley Hall includes a variety of activities, some of which are described briefly below.

Self-Care

Staff have been trained to identify the self-care tasks or parts of tasks each person can manage successfully.* The objective is for staff to do nothing for a resident that he/she can do him/herself, with the assumption that unnecessary assistance only increases dependence and implies that the elderly person is no longer capable. The self-care activities include brushing teeth, bathing, getting dressed and undressed, selecting clothes to wear, combing and brushing hair, shaving, applying make-up, and nail care. The extent to which residents can manage these tasks varies greatly. For example, if staff lay out the toothbrush and paste and remind them to brush their teeth, two of the residents are still able to pick up the toothbrush and press the toothpaste from a tube onto the brush, hold it under water, brush and rinse. Eight of the residents are able to do the necessary steps, if staff instruct them one step at a time and give occasional assistance. For one person, staff must apply the paste, put the brush in the individual's hand, turn on the faucet, help guide the hand to get water on the brush, and say "Now you are ready to brush your teeth." Staff then aid and instruct in the brushing and

---

*In its many projects, the Institute of Gerontology has used the technique of task breakdown in working with impaired elderly to allow for the various levels of complexity of a task and to compensate for the differing levels of competency. Each individual is given a part of the task to do which matches his/her level and type of competence.

rinsing. With much reminding, encouragement and assistance from staff, even the most impaired person in the project is still able to manage the actual brushing process.

Housekeeping Chores

With the permission of the State Department of Public Health, project staff were able to convert one of the small rooms into a kitchen, containing essential kitchen appliances and other items such as coffee maker, popcorn popper, ice cream maker, implements, and supplies. (In the context of rehabilitation, the Department uses the term "learning center" rather than "kitchen.") The Department also gave permission for the dishes to be done by residents in the kitchen. Although all meals are brought to the area from the central kitchen, residents often prepare a variety of snacks. Residents eat their noon and evening meals together in the small dining area. There is no scheduled time for breakfast, however, and residents come to the dining room whenever they get up, sometimes in their robes. This arrangement accommodates both the early risers and the late sleepers.

Both resident assistants and the housekeeper work with residents to enable them to continue a variety of tasks. They are involved in the following housekeeping chores: setting the tables, removing dishes from the table, washing and drying dishes, running the vacuum, baking and frosting muffins and cookies, making home-made ice cream, changing beds, folding towels, sweeping the kitchen floor, preparing vegetables for soup and fruit for special snacks, making sandwiches, and serving refreshments to guests. Several, with the guidance of staff, take responsibility for watering plants, feeding the canary, and putting feed in the outdoor window sill bird feeder.

Shared Activities

A number of activities have been introduced and tested involving small groups or all residents if they are interested. These activities have enriched the life on Wesley Hall while at the same time demonstrating the range of capacities still present in even very impaired persons.

a. Volunteer Activities

With the support and encouragement of staff members, most of the residents have been able to participate in carefully selected service projects. They frequently fold newsletters and flyers for the American Red Cross. Two or more residents may be involved in the completion of some tasks. For example, a flyer that requires two folds is too complex a task for most residents. The task is then broken down into two steps, with one person making the first fold and a second person completing the task.

Another popular service activity is preparing garnishes for the downstairs dining room. The dietary staff supply cherries, pineapple cubes, cheese cubes, ham cubes, olives, etc., and toothpicks. Residents assemble the canapés for Sunday night suppers in the large central dining room of the retirement home. They enjoy this activity, and there are many comments about the foods that should go together on a toothpick, and an occasional sampling of the items to be assembled.

b. Activities with Families and Children

Family potlucks have become a regular part of the life on Wesley Hall. Every three or four months families have been invited to attend, bring whatever food they wish, and meet together to learn about coming events and discuss their own concerns. A number of small tables arranged in the hallway enable families to share dinner with their relative. The occasion usually ends with a sing-a-long in which everyone participates.

Residents have been especially responsive to children when they visit the area. They have shared a variety of activities—making and frosting cupcakes, feeding the canary, and singing together. Parents of the children are prepared in advance about the goals of Wesley hall, how the children will be involved, and the behaviors of the children, such as running or shouting, that might be upsetting to the residents. The activities are carefully selected and structured so that the children and residents can share in a task. The visits usually end with refreshments and singing together.

c. Reminiscing

A number of small group activities have been centered around reminiscing. Individual posters have been made showing events in the resident's life. The staff person acting as group leader encourages each person to talk, as much as they are able, about whatever they can remember from their earlier life, and the posters are passed around for everyone to see. Some family members have prepared photograph albums with captions to identify relatives and friends or to explain the events. These, too, are used in the session.

Occasionally reminiscence centers around antique objects which residents can see and handle. Such items as a washboard, a button hook, an old-fashioned iron that had to be heated on the stove, etc., draw many comments and references to similar items they once owned. This activity was also effective in an earlier project with a severely impaired group of elderly persons who could no longer communicate verbally. When the items were introduced one woman placed her sweater on the table and began to iron it; another woman went through the motions of scrubbing clothes on the washboard.

d. Reading Group

Several residents are still able to read and they have enjoyed reading aloud to other residents. They are especially fond of humorous stories about children.

e. Handcrafts

Handcrafts, such as wall hangings for children's gifts or seasonal motifs to decorate a twig from a pussy willow tree, are done occasionally. The crafts are broken into a series of steps, e.g., tracing, cutting, and gluing, with each participant doing only the part he or she is able to manage successfully. This arrangement enables the group to produce a final product that is of good quality.

f. Humorous Activities

Because residents have responded so well to rather playful and humorous activities, staff have tested out a number of things to learn whether they would be appealing. Clowning has been especially successful as a means of entertaining both residents and visiting small children. On several occasions a resident assistant and a resident have put on clown make-up and costumes and moved from room to room sometimes doing an imitation of a soft shoe dance. Clowning was first tried as a part of a Halloween party when only staff and residents were present. It stimulated much laughter and comments, and parts of the costumes, including a bulbous red nose, were passed around and tried on by other residents. It should be noted that the approach used in initiating and presenting the clowning activity is critical. It is essential not to indicate disrespect for participants as adults. It can provide opportunities to reminisce about clowns and circuses and to discuss things that everyone has done to have fun throughout life.

The "hat activity," probably as much as any other, demonstrates the spontaneity and humor of residents. One of the resident assistants has a collection of hats, ranging from baseball cap to sombrero, to elaborate ones in various shapes and colors. The hats are passed from one to another and, with much laughter, residents try them on and view themselves in a mirror which the resident assistant has ready. This, as well as a number of other activities, has demonstrated the therapeutic value of humor and laughter. The *36-Hour Day* (Mace and Rabins, 1981) notes the retention of human emotions in persons with dementia in these words: "A dementing illness does not suddenly end a person's capacity to experience love or joy, nor does it end her ability to laugh. . . . Happiness may seem out of place in the face of trouble, but in fact it crops up unexpectedly."

Humor has played an important part in establishing the climate on Wesley Hall. It has been effective in raising the moods of residents and in helping them respond. The need for humor includes the need for silliness as well as subtle, witty, and dignified humor.

g. Spontaneous Activities

A number of activities are introduced spontaneously to reduce anxiety and tension. Singing is one of the most popular, and two of the residents often begin a song, even when staff are not in the room, and others join in.

Exercise sessions and nerf ball toss also create a light mood and almost all residents respond immediately when the activities are introduced by staff.

STAFF APPROACHES

Training for Wesley Hall teaches staff to identify the strengths and needs of each individual rather than to focus on problem behaviors. The goal is to learn how to recognize the remaining capacities and to build on them while, at the same time, accepting the individual's deficits and behaviors. To aid in the identification of competencies and deficits, Wesley Hall uses an individualized approach to assessment of each resident. Prior to selection, extensive interviews with residents and family members are conducted and at least one extended visit to the unit by the resident enables staff to observe and record the person's social and functional skills. Once an individual has been selected to live on the unit, further monitoring continues in order to keep abreast of changes in needs and functioning levels.

Wesley Hall has recently begun using neuropsychological assessment instruments specifically designed for people with dementia. They serve to alert staff to an individual's potential as well as to his or her degree of deterioration. Institute staff believe that neuropsychological assessments can play a valuable role in the development of intervention programming. It is difficult to avoid overestimating or underestimating an individual's abilities while guiding him or her through a particular task. With the help of systematic and detailed observations of the individual in the performance of a task and of standardized or adapted neuropsychological tests, the risk of frustrating a resident by making a task too difficult or too easy can be minimized. This enables a resident to successfully accomplish an activity and continue to grow even with the inevitably increasing impairment.

Staff on Wesley Hall have found that the *approach* they use will usually make the difference in their success or failure with an individual in any given situation. Therefore, Institute staff have developed a compendium of approaches from which staff can draw in their everyday interactions with residents.

The key to the success of these approaches is versatility. The approaches include gentle cajoling, affectionate encouragement, diversion, humor, withdrawing and returning later to try again when the resident's mood may be right, giving the resident time to think and respond, and varying the introduction of a topic that may trigger resistance (such as bathing).

Coercion, repetitive use of any specific approach, uniform approaches with all residents, and rigid routines and schedules were strongly discouraged in the staff training. Residents on Wesley Hall are a diverse group of people who seem to have a strong sense of individuality and personal identity. They are not subdued as are many of the elderly who have lived in institutions for years, and they are more active than most of the physically frail persons living in nursing homes. They resist the practices followed in many treatment settings. They become angry and sometimes combative when staff are controlling. They rebel against efforts to make them conform at the expense of their own individual preferences, a practice which essentially erases individuality in many nursing homes. Restraints have never been used, and sedatives or psychotropic drugs are used only rarely, and then for short periods of time.

Sundowning and Night Restlessness

Many approaches were tested out during the first three months of the project. During that period, night was almost as active as daytime. Most residents were up for long periods of time, at first wandering aimlessly from living room down the hall to the den and back again. The resident assistant who covered the night shift began to engage each of the people who wandered in a variety of activities—playing games, chatting, baking cookies, setting the table for breakfast—and as the weeks passed they seemed to become more relaxed, secure and at home in the area. They were probably more tired at night, too, because of the variety of activities they took part in daily. By the fifth month, most of those who had wandered were sleeping through the night except for occasional trips to the bathroom.

The evening hours, shortly after supper, however, continue to be a difficult time, and most of the shared activities now occur during that period. This is a particularly stressful time of day for many of the residents. A number of researchers have hypothesized the causes of nocturnal wandering and agitation. Hodge (1984) refers to the early study by D. E. Cameron (1941) which attributes night wandering to the interaction between darkness and memory deficit. Hodge believes, however, that this explanation ignores the social dimension, and that the social isolation which usually accompanies the onset of darkness, being in a bedroom alone, for example, may be a major cause.

Experience on Wesley Hall would support Hodge's premise. Involvement with other residents and staff seems to be reassuring. It also helps to divert residents from whatever the focus of their agitation might be. Staff also often sit with residents for a short time after they go to bed to help them relax and to remind them that the staff person is near by and will be checking in from time to time to see if they are sleeping well. These measures have been effective in reducing evening restlessness and sundowning.

Incontinence

In a study on incontinence in demented patients, Pollock and Liberman (1974) stress that this behavior is a multifaceted problem which needs the combined intervention of reinforcement, visual cues, and treatment of any urinary tract infections which may be present.

Hodge (1984) in discussing the problems of using behavioral programs with incontinent persons with dementia pointed out that it cannot be assumed

> that the patient has the neuropsychological capabilities necessary to be able to perform all the necessary steps required to achieve the target . . . it follows that any neuropsychological deficit which interferes with achieving the behavioral goal should be identified, and the means to overcome it, if this is possible, should be incorporated within the behavioral programme.

Four of the first residents who moved to Wesley Hall had been incontinent when they were living in the retirement home. The plan of interventions for the treatment of this group was multifaceted. Staff of the Incontinence Clinic** at the University of Michigan examined all residents shortly after admission to the area to determine if urinary tract infections were present. A number of the women had vaginal infections and were appropriately treated. For those who were incontinent, individualized toilet schedules were developed and followed throughout each 24 hours. On the recommendations of the staff of the Incontinence Clinic, liquid intake was greatly increased. Fruit juices were made available anytime. This additional intake not only provided the body with needed liquids but also filled the bladder sufficiently to give a clear message of the need to urinate.

In an effort to help direct residents to the location of the communal bathrooms, small colorful awnings were installed over the bathroom doors, red for women, blue for men. Frequent reminders by staff helped orient residents to the extent that occasionally a resident could be heard to tell another resident who was searching for a bathroom, "Go down to the red 'light'." Signs were also posted in the hallway pointing the direction to the bathrooms. Signs on the bathroom doors, planned to give additional visual cues, demonstrated the importance of appropriate terminology. The first sign attached, "Women," only increased confusion. Several would stand together at times reading the words and saying "What's that?" or other expressions indicating their confusion over the purpose of the room. The label was changed to read "Ladies' Bathroom," a term which had meaning to them.

As staff learned to know residents and their habits and moods, they became able to identify signals indicating a need to urinate. One man, for example, often sat quietly looking at a newspaper for long periods of time. Suddenly he would stand, look around the room in an uncertain way, and then begin to become agitated and angry. Staff learned to identify this as a signal that he needed to go to the bathroom. When staff immediately offered to walk with him to the bathroom door, they helped him avoid incontinence as well as the anger which had occurred earlier. Of the four residents who were

---

**Staff of the Incontinence Clinic included Dr. Thelma Wells and Carol Brink.

incontinent at the beginning of the project, three responded to treatment to the extent that two were no longer incontinent and the third had only occasional problems.

Anxiety Reactions

It soon became apparent that residents were very sensitive and reactive to the actions of other residents and staff. Moods could shift quickly and for no apparent reason, and in the first few months staff were constantly attempting to cope with the agitation and combativeness over which residents had no control.

Staff soon learned that insisting on baths, for example, could draw much resistance and anger. Attempts at "reasoning" only aggravated the situation. Now staff sit and chat with a resident who has been resistive in the past, then suggest they walk down the hall together, then casually suggest they walk into the bathroom. A hot tub has been prepared in advance, and the staff person talks about how good a warm bath will feel. This often helps the resident accept the bath. The unhurried, undemanding, calm and light approach is usually the most effective. Some residents refuse the first time and even the second, but accept the third time without resistance. Staff are convinced now that it sometimes takes residents that long to comprehend what they are being asked to do.

Occasionally a resident may become very angry if there is too much commotion or too many people in the area. The change of mood may be expressed by a sudden burst of profanity or yelling. Staff are often able to calm a resident when they sense a change by suggesting a walk together down the hall or that they share some fruit juice together in the kitchen. The mood usually passes quickly and the resident is able to return to the group.

A CASE PROFILE

Hannah has been a resident of Wesley Hall since it first opened in December of 1983. She has a diagnosis of Alzheimer's disease accompanied by depression for which she is being treated with medication. Her case profile is very briefly presented here.

Hannah's behaviors and performance on a variety of neuropsychological tests have been assessed at intervals over a 12-month period. These behaviors and test scores suggest Hannah's impairment is quite severe, and that she does indeed have a major organic component (i.e., brain pathology) to her disorder. She is also depressed. Her scores on the Mental Status Questionnaire by Kahn et al. (1960) have consistently been 8 to 10 errors placing her in the category of the severely impaired with the other residents on the unit. Her initial score on the Isaacs and Kennie Set Test (1973) naming colors, animals, towns, and fruit, was 14 out of a possible 40, placing her slightly below the group's average initial score of 17. Hannah's subsequent scores on the Set Test dropped to 6 over a twelve-month period. Errors on the last four trials on Green and Fink's (1954) Face-Hand Test have been consistently high. Her score on Folstein et al. (1975) Mini-Mental State was 7 out of a possible 30 points.

These scores as well as her performance on other neuropsychological tests indicate that Hannah is severely aphasic, which is particularly evident in her frequent use of words which do not accurately convey her intended meaning, e.g., "Are you the dressmaker?" when she means "hairdresser." Hannah is often aware of these errors and is embarrassed by them.

Although Hannah is aphasic, she also relies heavily on verbal techniques to complete an unfamiliar task. For example, when copying a simple design she "talks her way through it" step by step. This reliance on verbal skills, with the accompanying aphasia, presents a challenge to staff when presenting Hannah with a new job to learn.

Hannah exhibits many competencies. For example, she does write simple sentences; she can read directional signs; and she has excellent right-left and personal body orientation. She appears to see and recognize items in all parts of her visual field, and she can identify objects and colors accurately. Hannah also still recognizes herself in the mirror. She does not confuse the image with the real object, and she can locate a real object by seeing its reflection in the mirror.

Hannah's deficits include great difficulty in consciously re-

calling events from long ago and recently. She has more difficulty learning unfamiliar tasks than do some of the other
residents. Hannah's appreciation of spatial relationships, particularly in tasks where she must construct something, is quite
impaired. Her spatial orientation in terms of the larger physical environment is still relatively intact, although because of
her poor memory, she often forgets where the bathroom is.

Hannah seems to have great difficulty generating an abstract picture in her mind, such as the order of tasks to be
done to complete an activity. For example, she stands in the
kitchen for a short while after a meal, seeming to sense that
something comes next, but does not volunteer to do the
dishes. If someone asks her to help with dishes or if she sees
the sink being filled with water or dishes being stacked in
preparation for washing dishes, she readily begins washing. If
there are no obvious suggestions of dish washing, she stands
uncertainly for a moment and then proceeds to her room.

Probably Hannah's strongest asset is her appreciation of
social interaction. She does love to be with people, if she feels
competent among them, and she enjoys a good laugh. In spite
of her blunted emotional expressions and her depression, she
frequently can be cajoled with humor and affection into doing
something. Her performance on any task usually improves
dramatically with her mood.

Hannah had lived most of her married life in the town
where the retirement home housing Wesley Hall is located.
She began having severe memory problems shortly before the
death of her husband, and after his death, soon moved to the
retirement home when her son realized she was unable to live
alone. Her son describes Hannah as being a very social person who enjoyed people, but he feels that the move to Wesley
Hall has brought out the humor and spontaneity in his
mother.

She had great difficulty adjusting to the large retirement
home. Staff frequently found her wandering around both day
and night searching for her husband. Only with the help of
hall neighbors was she able to find the large central dining
room or the hall's bathroom. As her disorientation increased
her neighbors in the retirement home found the reponsibility
of helping her overwhelming, and they seemed relieved to see
her move to Wesley Hall.

Hannah was one of the first of the eleven residents to move to the area. By that time Wesley Hall staff had become well acquainted with her, for part of the staff training in preparation for the project was to spend time with each of the residents and to learn to know them as individuals. As she became relaxed with them, her humor and whimsical responses became a regular part of their conversations together.

Hannah has participated in most of the activities on the unit. She can dress and undress herself with step by step reminders from staff. This consists primarily of reminding her what the next item of clothing is to put on, and what the overall goal is (i.e., undressing versus dressing). She is capable of accomplishing such tasks as determining the front versus the back of her nightgown, which she usually does without prompting, and of knowing the implication of that in terms of actually putting the nightgown on.

Two of her favorite activities are group singing and ball tossing. At times, when she resists getting up from bed, staff have learned that stepping to the door of her room, tossing a nerf ball in her direction and saying, "We need you for a ball game" will be sufficient to lure her to the living room. When she appears she immediately begins to toss the ball to someone in the room.

When a clowning program was implemented to entertain small children who visited the area, Hannah responded with enthusiasm when invited to don make-up and clown costume. She fell naturally into the role and obviously enjoyed the reactions of the children.

The most difficult time of day for Hannah is early evening when she begins to search anxiously for her deceased husband. She insists that he is coming to pick her up, and becomes quite agitated if staff do not intervene. It is the policy of Wesley Hall not to confront residents with reality when they insist, as in Hannah's case, that someone, long deceased, is still a part of their world. Staff have found that such a direct approach only causes the individual to grieve, and increases agitation. Instead staff use supportive affection or diversions, such as changing topics or activities, in an effort to shift the focus to something to which the resident usually responds. Hannah is very fond of her son, and when she begins to search for her husband, staff will walk with her and begin to talk with her about the last visit her son, Frank, made and the things they did together. She usually asks, "Was he here?" The staff person continues to talk about the good time they had together and her mood changes and her agitation decreases. Staff then walks with her to her room and explains that this is where she lives now. She often denies this, but gradually accepts it, as her furniture, the picture on the wall of Frank and his family, and a bouquet of silk flowers he brought her are pointed out to her. She is fascinated by the flowers and always remarks about their beauty and freshness even though she has never watered them. On one of his visits, her son wrote a note with a felt pen on a large piece of white paper and fastened it to her closet door. He wrote about what a good time they had had together, how much he loved her, and how pleased he was that she was living in her new home. Staff points this out to Hannah, and she reads it over carefully. This reassurance enables her to relax and prepare for bed, and she quickly falls asleep.

Many of the intervention strategies used with Hannah have been identified or alluded to in the text of this paper and in the description of her case profile above. These include the notes written by her son, the gentle joking and singing to encourage her to attempt a task, the anticipation of an upcoming job or event by telling her about it a few minutes beforehand, the diversion technique used when she is agitated, the availability of environmental clues to remind or instruct her regarding an activity such as dishwashing, as well as many others. A few specific applications of neuropsychological and behavioral assessments in developing interventions will be briefly noted here.† Most of these interventions are already used in many treatment settings.

Because Hannah can identify objects and colors, coding the physical environment with color or decorations to orient her is appropriate for her. Staff do not need to avoid presenting items to her on either side of her body, because she can generally see and recognize all items in her visual field. This,

---

†A deeper and more detailed analysis of this case and its illustration of the application of neuropsychological assessment to development of intervention strategies is in preparation.

along with her relatively intact personal body orientation and environmental spatial organization, noted above, means simple verbal instructions can be quite useful, and excessive demonstration unnecessary, when she is dressing or setting the table. The mirror is sometimes useful to her in dressing, because she still recognizes herself in the mirror and can locate reflected objects such as the arm and neck holes in her dresses.

Sensitivity to the embarrassment she experiences when she has difficulty in finding words usually results in subtle aid from staff in conversations and in approaches. Comments rather than questions are initiated by staff. They usually request opinions rather than facts from her, and use short simple sentences and nonverbal communication techniques (Bartol, 1979).

Hannah needs time to accomplish anything. She needs time to hear, to think, to get motivated, to execute an action. Therefore, staff must talk slowly with her and wait patiently for her responses. When Hannah is required to produce names or facts, which is difficult for her, the requests for information are interspersed with non-threatening conversation.

Wesley Hall staff recognized that Hannah's behaviors must be seen in the context of Hannah's own history and personality, as well as in the context of the specific physical, social, and emotional environments in which they occur. Therefore, "problem behaviors" are not addressed independent of Hannah herself. When a "problem behavior" or a deficit is identified in Hannah, the context in which it occurs is always assessed: when, where, why, with whom, and how does the behavior or deficit become apparent or troublesome. Frequently staff determine that the focus for the intervention must be the environment (physical, social, or emotional) and not necessarily simply Hannah herself.

For this reason, the general ambience of Wesley Hall is attended to. Hannah thrives in an almost party-like atmosphere. Staff concentrate on creating situations which are socially stimulating and fun. Hugs and joking are very effective, not only in encouraging her to do tasks she may resist doing, but also in increasing her skill performance and the success with which she learns new tasks.

For Hannah an important strength is her appreciation of

friends. Her ready laugh and willingness to engage in a fun, group activity which does not demand more of her than she can produce, contribute much to the enjoyment of other residents and staff. It is generally assumed on Wesley Hall that if you want to have a good time, Hannah will be there to join in.

CONCLUSION

Without question, persons with Alzheimer's disease represent a very special group of people for whom our current care system is neither prepared to accommodate nor equipped to respond to their special needs. Direct service staff need guidance and instruction in helping residents with dementia to continue to care for themselves to the extent possible. It is often difficult for untrained staff to determine what capacities still remain or the amount of assistance the impaired resident needs to be successful in a given task. Physical and occupational therapists can, and in many instances have, become key persons in enriching intervention programs by developing functional assessment tools and intervention strategies for this vulnerable group who are living in residential and nursing home settings. As models and instructors, these professionals can help the direct service staff become more effective in working with the mentally impaired elderly. What is needed is a creative urge to design and test new interventions that will help sustain the older person's capabilities, minimize her/his deficits, and provide a quality of life that is rewarding and fulfilling.

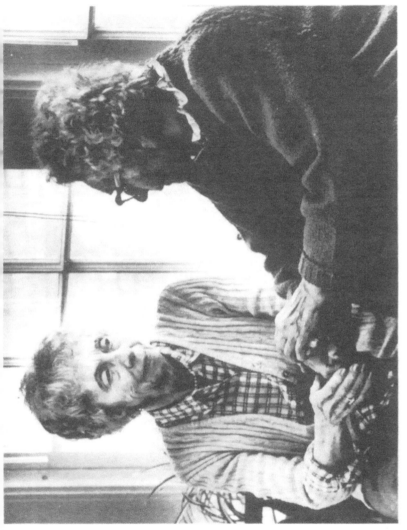

FIGURE 1. Two friends share a moment together.

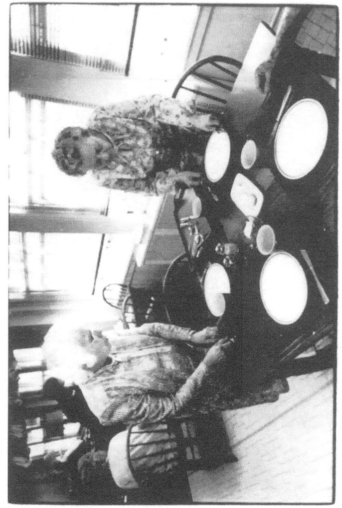

FIGURE 2. Residents help with household tasks such as setting the tables.

REFERENCES

Bartol, M. A. Nonverbal communication in patients with Alzheimer's disease. *Journal of Gerontological Nursing*, 1979, 5, 4, 21–31, July-August.

Brody, E. M., Cole, C., & Moss, M. Individualizing therapy for the mentally impaired aged. *Social Casework*, 1973, October, 453–461.

Cameron, D. E. Studies in senile nocturnal delirium. *Psychiatric Quarterly*, 1941, 15, 47–53.

Coons, D. H. The therapeutic milieu. In W. Reichel, M.D. (Ed.) *Clinical Aspects of Aging*. Baltimore: Williams and Wilkins, 1983.

Folstein, M. F., Folstein, S. E., & McHugh, P. R. Mini-mental state: a practical method for grading the cognitive state of patients for the clinician. *Journal of Psychiatric Research*, 1975, 12, 189–198.

Green, M. & Fink, M. Standardization of the Face-Hand Test. *Neurology*, 1954, 4, 211.

Haugen, P. K. Behavior of patients with dementia. *Danish Medical Bulletin*, 1985, 32, Supplement No. 1, 62–65.

Hellebrandt, F. A. Comment: the senile dement in our midst. *The Gerontologist*, 1978, 18, 1, 67–70.

Hodge, J. Towards behavioural analysis of dementia. In I. Hanley and J. Hodge (Eds.) *Psychological Approaches to the Care of the Elderly*. London and Sydney: Croom Helm Australia Pty. Ltd., 1984.

Isaacs, B. & Kennie, A. T. The Set Test as an aid to the detection of dementia in old people. *British Journal of Psychiatry*, 1973, 132, 467–470.

Kahn, R. L., Goldfarb, A. I., Pollack, M., & Peck, A. Brief objective measures for the determination of mental status in the aged. *American Journal of Psychiatry*, 1960, 117, 326–328.

Loftus, E. F. *Memory*. Reading, MA: Addison-Wesley Publishing Company, 1980.

Mace, N. L. & Rabins, P. V. *The 36-Hour Day*. Baltimore: The Johns Hopkins University Press, 1981.

Pollack, D. D. & Liberman, R. P. Behavior therapy of incontinence in demented inpatients. *The Gerontologist*, 1974, 14, 6, 488–491.

Woods, R. T. & Britton, P. G. *Clinical Psychology and the Elderly*. Rockville: Aspen Systems Corporation, 1985.

REFERENCES

An Eclectic Group Program for Nursing Home Residents with Dementia

Charlotte Campbell Maloney, OTR,
Terran Daily, OTR

ABSTRACT. This paper describes the rationale used in the design of a group treatment program for elderly residents with a diagnosis of dementia or organic brain syndrome who lived in a residential center offering multiple levels of care from independent living to skilled nursing care. The selection process and general approach are discussed. The assessment procedure is outlined and the meeting format described. General results of the project are provided. Possible avenues for further investigation are identified.

Disoriented, sensory impaired residents appeared to present insoluble programming challenges to the social service staff at Jewish Home for the Aged, San Francisco. Cognitively impaired individuals, who also demonstrated significant hearing and/or vision losses, appeared unable to benefit from group programs offered within the Activity Program. The

---

Charlotte Maloney is a staff occupational therapist at Sacred Heart General Hospital, Eugene, Oregon. Terran Daily is a staff occupational therapist at Alta Bates–Herrick Rehabilitation Center, Berkeley, California. Successively, each was the director of the Sensory Awareness Training Project, Jewish Home for the Aged, San Francisco, California. The authors thank the following individuals whose support made the Sensory Awareness Training Project possible: Howard Lader, LCSW, former Director of Social Services; Jerry Levine, Executive Director; Gertrude McDonnell, RN, Director of Nursing Services; Marion Kingsbury, RN, Director of Inservice Education; each nurse and nurses' aide of Second West and 2A units; Gregory Hughes; and Miriam Singer-Breyer, MS. Jim Maloney and Noah Potkin are thanked for their technical assistance in the writing of this paper. Readers are asked to address correspondence to the authors c/o Occupational Therapy Department, Sacred Heart General Hospital, 1200 Hilyard Street, Eugene, OR 97440.

55

ability to provide ongoing one-to-one programming was impossible due to the staffing and funding constraints faced by all agencies serving institutionalized elderly.

Jewish Home retained a gerontic occupational therapist with interest and experience in serving chronically impaired elderly to direct a pilot project exploring group program options for these residents. The pilot project was to explore whether sensory stimulation activities in a group treatment format might reverse or prevent further cognitive decline. The project was named The Sensory Awareness Training Project (referred to as the SP in this paper).

The job description of the SP Director included developing and conducting assessments of each group member, developing and implementing a group treatment format, assessing the effectiveness of such a format, determining whether some aspects of the program could be implemented by other staff, maintaining records and supplies, and writing quarterly progress reports. Two responsibilities were added later—offering practicum experiences to interested university students and providing in-service instruction to members of the activity and nursing staffs.

BASIC DECISIONS

Two distinct types of residents needed a group activity. The disoriented person with physical limitations, requiring maximum nursing care, was differentiated from the partially oriented or easily confused resident, requiring less nursing care. To promote optimal group dynamics, two separate meeting groups were formed. Group members for the less impaired were selected from several nursing units; each member was at least partially oriented to time/place/person and had varying degrees of sensory and motor loss. These group meetings lasted approximately one hour. The group of the more impaired residents was composed of members from the maximum care nursing section of Jewish Home; each was disoriented and presented with significant physical limitations. Depending upon the responsiveness of the members during the session, these meetings lasted one-half to three-quarters of an hour.

The overall objective of the groups was to provide sensory stimulation activities in order to maximize the use of each resident's remaining sensory channels, prevent a state of sensory deprivation which can occur during age related sensory losses (Carroll, 1978) (Byron, 1978) and facilitate the maximum functional level of each group member (in communication, cognitive, social and self care skills). The goal of the Maintenance Group (less impaired residents) was to prevent or slow decline in skills, while the goal of the Intervention Group (more impaired residents) was to change behavior. Increases in social behavior such as initiation and participation in conversation, smiling, making eye contact, level of alertness, awareness of self and environment, participation in self care, and cognitive functions (such as memory and reasoning) were sought.

The size of each group was limited to six residents. Meetings were three times per week and were conducted by a group leader and a maximum of two assistants. Most often the leader was the SP Director, assisted by one student volunteer. A minimum time commitment of three months was required of each student assistant. They were occupational therapy, psychology, and gerontology students desiring experience with cognitively impaired older adults. The orientation of each student included training in the SP general approach in order to ensure continuity in experience for the group members.

Group meetings were structured like informal "get-to-gethers." A teatime or coffee klatch atmosphere was created by the language and attitude of the assistants and leader. Meetings were held in the day room of the nursing unit. Attendees sat in a circle. Usually, wheelchairbound residents were assisted into day room chairs; the purpose of this was to create sufficient proximity for residents to touch and hear one another. Group members' positions in the circle were determined by which sensory deficits had been identified in their pretest. For example, the members with the most hearing impairments were seated beside the group leader, while residents with visual limitations were seated next to an assistant or the leader, who provided verbal and tactile cues in group activities.

ASSESSMENT

In assessing the needs of the residents to be served, an assessment tool was devised. (See Assessment Data Sheet and Assessment Protocol in Appendix.) SP group members were assessed in the following areas of function: sensory perception, memory, orientation, activities of daily living, attention span, posture, strength, range of motion, eye contact, insight, following directions, body awareness, muscle tone, quality of movement, equilibrium responses, trunk rotation, and ocular pursuits. The data for activity level and self care function were obtained from the daily nursing care notes in the medical record. Mental status and cognitive function were assessed by interview, during which clinical observations were also noted. Sensory perception status was then assessed. The remainder of the procedure was completed in two sessions as the resident tolerated. An abbreviated form of this assessment procedure was utilized for the assessments of all six of the original Intervention Group members due to fatigue and attention span limitations. Maintenance Group members tolerated the length of the full procedure.

Group members were reassessed at six month intervals. In addition to results obtained from the assessment procedure, clinical observations were recorded in three methods. The SP Director completed weekly notes of observations made during one-to-one and group interactions. Nursing staff completed the Ward Behavior Rating Scale, while activity program and SP staff completed the Group Behavior Scale. These two scales were adapted from the work of Kiernat (1978) and rated behaviors such as facial expression, attentiveness, initiation/participation in conversation, attention to personal appearance (grooming/hygiene skills), interest in activities, and appropriate social behavior. Assessment results and behavioral observations were the basis for measuring change throughout the project.

GENERAL APPROACH

The general approach consisted of a philosophy which influenced every interaction with each SP group member. The characteristics of this approach were: respect for each resident's wisdom, life experience and individuality; non-judgmental; non-parental; affectionate; friendly; warm; genuine interest in the resident; respectful of each resident's choice, including the choice not to attend all or part of SP meetings; expectation of appropriate behavior ("I like you but I dislike your behavior" to inappropriate behavior); appreciative of the expression of feelings while avoiding any pressure upon group members to express feelings; recognition that each time a resident participated in conversation or in an activity, they had made an effort to communicate beyond barriers created by their sensory loss(es). This approach was maintained regardless of the resident's behavior. This general attitude guided every interaction with each resident from initial introduction, through pretesting and retesting, as well as during, before, and after group meetings.

Each resident was individually greeted and physically assisted to the meeting place by an SP staff person. This pre-meeting interaction was characterized by warmth and physical contact. Patting the resident's arm or holding hands while ambulating to the meeting place conveyed a genuine personal interest. Moreover, it was thought that this tactile stimulus might also alert the drowsy resident and calm the anxious resident. SP staff were sensitive to each resident's tolerance of this physical contact. Of the 16 residents who participated in SP groups over its three year span, only two appeared "tactilely defensive." This was similar to tactilely defensive behavior in learning disabled children reported by Ayres (1978). SP staff limited physical contact with these residents to holding or shaking hands and pats on the shoulder or upper back. With the majority of the SP group members, this physical contact evolved into hugging and/or walking or sitting arm-in-arm.

FRAMES OF REFERENCE

Elements from the work of various authors were blended into the design of the group meetings. The following identifies which concepts were influential and describes how the selected methods were utilized.

Reality Orientation vs. Validation

It was the design of the SP groups to reinforce each resident's identity as a mature adult possessing wisdom gained from life experience. Therefore, the formal classroom reality orientation model was replaced by the "twenty-four hour" style orientation as described by Byron (1978). SP staff responded to inaccurate statements by commenting "Does it seem like that to you?" after Feil's Validation/Fantasy approach (1980).

Orientation to the usual time, place, or current president was never emphasised. Instead, the group leader made general reference to the time of day (morning, afternoon), the season of the year, upcoming or current holiday (religious and national), place (Jewish Home and San Francisco), and names of group members (at each meeting each attendee wore first name only name tags). Current events or other specific orientation information were only pursued when a resident asked specific questions. This was regarded as a request for orientation. Rarely did group discussion develop from orienting statements.

Reminiscing

The rationale for the use of reminiscence is based upon Ebersole's chapter, "A Theoretical Approach to the Use of Reminiscence" (Burnside, 1978). Following her thinking, psychotherapeutic interpretation was not attempted. Reminiscing was facilitated during SP meetings as a method for group members, who otherwise were passive and uninvolved in their surroundings, to interact with peers by recalling past events. It was thought that minimally, storytellers would receive pleasure and increased self esteem from contributing to the group. It was hoped that the listeners would gain a sense of contact with others and a lessening of a sense of isolation by identifying with the feelings and experiences of their peers.

All activities in the group meetings were used as a springboard to reminisce. While residents handled the sensory stimuli objects, the group leader and assistants asked questions such as "What does this make you think of?" or "Have you ever seen/eaten/used anything like this before?" When a group member answered such questions, other residents were encouraged to share their reactions. Occasionally, the main group activity became reminiscing discussions. Sometimes reminiscing did not occur.

Remotivation Therapy

A basic format was sought to provide a sense of continuity for residents and to simplify the staff's planning of meetings. The steps of a meeting and the selection of a meeting theme were borrowed from Remotivation Therapy and modified for use in the SP. The Remotivation Therapy focus upon the world of work was replaced in the SP with a focus upon awareness of the self and the immediate environment. Some meetings triggered discussions of role(s) of group members, such as that role of spouse, parent, worker, or retiree. Other than this, there was no relationship between the focus of SP and Remotivation groups.

The steps of a Remotivation Therapy group (Robinson, per Ebersole in Burnside, 1978) were listed as: first, introductions/greetings; second, "bridge to reality" by reading an article; third, "sharing the world" discussion of the article with the use of visual aids and props; fourth, "appreciation of the world" discussion of the topic presented in the article and fostering each group member thinking about work in relation to themselves; and last, "climate of appreciation" phase of expressing pleasure in the group having met and of scheduling the next meeting. The first and last steps were incorporated into the SP format.

In the SP's modification of the three middle steps, they became one step. During this single middle step each resident handled and reacted to the sensory stimulation object(s). In many meetings, this led to reminiscing, as described above. The general concepts of "bridge to reality," "sharing the world," and "appreciation of the world" were used only in the phrasing of the presentation of sensory stimulation objects. The context of the presentation was social, that is, the way one would share a discovery with a peer.

In using the theme planning concept, SP themes were selected to serve as a link between sensory stimuli rather than as a link between group members and the work world. An example was selecting the theme of summer for sequentially presenting an arrangement of brightly colored, fresh flowers;

glasses of iced tea, and slices of fresh peach on a plate. Another example was the theme of summer vacation for the presentation of a strong smelling piece of seaweed, a color *National Geographic* photograph of sunbathers at a beach, a bucket of sand with two or three small objects "lost" in the sand, and glasses of ice and water.

Sensory Stimulation/Sensory Integration

Sensory stimulation was defined as the treatment approach by which single or multiple stimuli exciting a specific sensory channel (tactile, auditory, visual, olfactory, gustatory, or vestibular) was presented with the goal of increasing the acuity of that sense or of eliciting a generalized response such as an increased level of alertness (Richman, 1969) (Huber, 1973), reverse "senile" behavior patterns associated with age related sensory loss (Byron, 1978) (Carroll, 1978), and increase social and self care skills (Ross and Burdick, 1978 and 1981).

For use in the SP, sensory integration treatment approach was defined as the introduction of selected sensory stimuli, presented in a subcortical fashion with the goal of improving neurological organization and increasing both the number and quality of motor responses (Ayres, 1978). An example of presenting a sensory stimulus on a subcortical level in the SP was to offer members a bottle of scented body lotion and ask members whether they wished to use some on their hands. A purely cortical approach would have been to present the same fragrance in a container with the instruction, "Smell this, please," or "Can you identify this scent?" The difference was that had the resident been asked to process the act of inhaling the scent in and of itself, the main process would be registering the sensory input in cortical areas. Whereas, when asked to use the lotion with no instruction to identify or attend to the scent, conscious attention was focused upon the motor act of using the lotion and the olfactory input was thought to be processed at a subcortical level of the brain. It has been hypothesized that activities which take place on a subcortical level facilitate maximal integration of the sensory input (Ayres, 1978). It was assumed that the sensory input was being integrated when the motor responses such as eye contact, participation in conversation, passing the container to the next attendee, communicative gesturing, smiling, and following of instructions were observed. The success of Wavrick (1972) in using sensory integration techniques in treatment of residents with chronic brain syndrome, primary and secondary diagnosis, was noted.

Using these two overlapping approaches in SP meetings, activities were planned to stimulate each sensory channel during every meeting. Olfaction was the first sensory mode stimulated because of its neural connection to the potent reticular activating system, which was thought to be the center for arousal (Fox, 1966). Length of time in the first activity was determined by degree of response. The drowsier the residents, the longer the time spent. The next activity planned included tactile, visual and vestibular components. If lengthy discussion developed, then some planned activities were deleted. The last sensory activity of each session was gustatory in nature; taste activities seemed to serve as a "reward" for attending the meeting. The taste activity was considered multisensory because eating most foods provided simultaneous stimulation to olfactory, tactile (stereognosis, deep pressure or light touch, and/or temperature), and visual systems as well as the gustatory system.

It was thought that multiple sensory input was integrated better than single stimuli and that the multiple stimuli needed to be related to the same aspect of the environment (Ayres, 1978). It was likewise believed that self applied stimulation was more completely integrated into the nervous system than the same stimuli applied by another and that visual spatial perception was probably promoted by the processing of the sensory feedback from self-produced movement (Ayres, 1978). The SP modus operandi was to present multisensory stimuli and to construct activities requiring residents to manipulate, smell, see, and/or hear the object before moving it in some way and passing it to the member beside them.

MEETING FORMAT

The outline followed in each SP group session has been summarized in Figure 1. Every meeting followed the order of opening, introducing a theme, presenting activities relating to

FIGURE 1. SP FORMAT: ACTIVITY DESCRIPTIONS

BASIC ACTIVITY	VARIATIONS	COMMENTS
INTRODUCTIONS. Using large print name tags, leader introduces each person in turn.	1. Beginning with leader, each member introduces self with first and last names. 2. Each member introduces person on their right or left.	In higher level groups, name tags without verbal introductions may be enough once members know each other. Exception: visitor or new member in group.
CONVERSATION. Leader brings up topic and encourages group participation.	Weather, season, holidays, theme for the day (ocean, picnic, work, families, etc.), special happenings for group members.	Keep conversation on adult level. Elicit response from each member when possible. Encourage interaction among members and reminiscence.
SMELL. Pass around object or substance to be smelled.	Flowers, spices, perfumes, essential oils, flavorings, vinegar, horseradish, pine needles, etc. Avoid substances harmful if inhaled or spilled: ammonia, cinnamon oil.	Ask each person to respond to object or substance in some way: Do they like it? What does it remind them of? *Not* necessarily what is it? Can be hard to identify. Have members pass objects independently—spillage is rare.
TOUCH. Pass object with interesting texture or shape to look at and feel.	1. Rocks, shells, feathers, jewelry, brushes, scrubbers, sponges, fabrics, leaves, cooking utensils, tools. 2. Two or more contrasting objects: heavy-light, rough-smooth, hard-soft. 3. Hide object in box or bag and identify by touch alone. 4. Bury object in textured substance: rice, dried beans, cornmeal, sand. 5. Treasure hunt. Bury several coins or other attractive small objects in large tray of sand. How many objects can each person find in a specified time? 6. Hand lotion, lip balm, washing face and hands, massage, combing hair, filing nails.	Ask for response to object: What is it? How does it feel? Have you seen anything like it? Encourage reminiscence.
MOVEMENT. 1. Toss object from person to person.	Large balloon (soft and moves slowly, giving participant time to visually focus and prepare to hit or catch), beach ball, nerf ball, foam frisbee, bean bag.	Games are more involving and enjoyable than repetitive exercises, and as meaningful activity, may be more integrating to nervous system. (Ayers, 197)

FIGURE 1 (continued)

MOVEMENT.

2. Toss object into center.	Plastic horseshoes or rings onto stake. Beanbags into basket, box or hula hoop.	Neck exercises are an exception as they provide such direct stimulation to the semi-circular canals.
3. Parachute games.	All members hold and ripple parachute, or bounce ball or balloon in center of parachute.	
4. Moving to music.		
5. Neck exercises.	Move head up and down, right and left, ears to shoulders, in full circle. *Discontinue if dizziness results.*	

BREATH ACTIVITIES.

1. Blow pinwheel, party blowers, bubbles.		Singing is especially enjoyable and a good source of reminiscence.
2. Singing.		Bubble liquid may stain clothing

MOTOR PLANNING ACTIVITIES.	Rhythm band, clapping games, Simon says, "Mirrors"—each person copies leader's motions.	Motor planning is a complex capacity, requiring cooperation of sensory and motor systems. Often disturbed in neurologically impaired elders.
	Participants can take turns being leader.	Activities may need to be very simple.

TASTE.

1. Pass food to be tasted.	Cookies (distinct flavors such as chocolate chip, coconut, or gingersnap), candy (strong flavors—cinammon, peppermint or lemon), fruit, pickles, olives, crackers, pretzels, juice, ice cream, herb teas, coffee, beer, wine, liqueurs (in small amounts and with doctor's permission).	Watch for dietary restrictions: sugar, salt, allergies, dysphagia or puree diets.
	Contrast sweet, sour, bitter, salty, warm, cold, soft, crunchy, etc.	
2. Cooking class. Entire session is devoted to cooking.	Cookies, strawberry shortcake, ice cream sundaes, mashed potatoes, salads —fruit, vegetable, egg or fish.	Cooking is a good holiday or seasonal activity. Also makes a good birthday party. Have all ingredients ready and a recipe in large print. Give participants jobs they are capable of and help when needed. Preparing half the batch ahead of time and cooking it while the group prepares the second half prevents a long waiting period while the food cooks. Waiting time can be used for singing, balloon toss, etc.

the theme, and closing. But the length of the meeting and length of the steps was determined by the group dynamic on the given day.

SUPPLIES

Supplies used for the SP meetings were as varied as possible. Since many stimulus objects are "found," rather than purchased, the expense of many activities was only the staff time spent obtaining them. (See Figure 2 for the list of supplies used.)

Figure 2.   LIST OF SUPPLIES

```
BASIC

    Name tags
    Essential oils
    Spices
    Perfumes
    Body lotions, various scents
    Lip balm
    Large combs (one for each person, or disinfect between uses)
    Nail files
    Unbreakable hand mirror
    Fabric scraps, various textures
    Nature objects: rocks, shells, feathers, driftwood
    Containers of various sizes: bowls, wash basin, empty milk jugs, sheet cake pan
    Dried grains and beans: rice, buckwheat, corn, lentils, limas, oatmeal, etc.
    Small objects to bury: pennies, thimbles, rings, buttons, birthday candles, etc.
    Familiar objects for stereognosis: kitchen utensils, tools, office items, grooming
        implements.
    Bag or box for hiding objects
    Beach ball
    Bean bags
    Pinwheels
    Party blowers
    Large balloons (available from Fred Sammons, Inc., Box 32, Brookfield IL 60513-0032.)
    Parachute (available from Army surplus store or Flaghouse, Inc., 18 W 18th St.,
        New York NY 10011.)
    Rhythm instruments (can be homemade)


OPTIONAL

    Radio, record or cassette player
    Hand held communication device for hearing impaired ("One-to-One Communicator" from
        One-to-One Communications, 678 W. Cedar St., Olathe KS 66061, or "Listening Aid
        System" from Radio Shack, catalogue numbers 33-1091/33-1000.  Others are avail-
        able--consult an audiologist for further information.)


EXPENDABLE

    Foods:  salty, sweet, sour, bitter
    Beverages:  hot, cold, various tastes
    Nature objects:  flowers, leaves, snow
```

RESULTS

Over the three year course of the project, membership was fairly constant. Two members of the Maintenance Group died and two Intervention Group members were terminated. Termination of membership occurred when a participant consistently declined in function over a period of a minimum of twelve months or became so disruptive as to interfere with the process of group meetings. New members replaced those who were deceased or terminated, making a total of sixteen participants in the project. (See Figure 3 for identifying characteristics of each group member.)

No statistical analysis was attempted with the results because the SP was a pilot project, not a controlled study. The conclusions offered are presented as general indications for further study and for trial use by clinicians. The most concrete outcomes of this pilot project were the development of the assessment tool and the integration of group treatment techniques for the population served. General observations of residents' responses to types of stimuli and a gross analysis of the final assessment data were made.

General Observations of Group Leaders

During group meetings, several observations of general group responses were noted. Sensory stimuli were found to be easily integrated into group activities. Providing a social context in which the stimuli were introduced appeared to facilitate their acceptance by residents. An example was the incorporation of strong, non-irritating olfactory stimuli into multisensory activities such as baking or eating selected foods or sharing a scented body lotion. Another example was creating guessing games for tactile stimuli, such as placing common objects in a bag filled with a grain or beans or such as placing one object in a roomy paper bag and having residents guess the name of the object.

A high level of response was noted to tactile stimuli included in touching and hugging residents. A favorite activity was neck rubs in pairs, lotion was incorporated at times, while quick tapping replaced massaging during other meetings. The physical contact between residents and SP staff (discussed

Figure 3. IDENTIFYING CHARACTERISTICS OF SP PARTICIPANTS.
Age and years in Home are as of entry into SP Project. Evaluation Outcome is expressed as positive changes/negative changes from initial to final evaluations.

RESIDENT	SEX	AGE	DIAGNOSIS	YEARS IN HOME	MONTHS IN PROJECT	EVAL OUTCOME	CLINICAL OBSERVATIONS
A	F	92	CBS	4.0	36	4+/1-	Decr. tactile defensiveness
B	F	88	senile psychosis	8.0	24 terminated	0+/8-	Incr. incontinence & withdrawal
C	F	89	CBS	8.5	36	4+/1-	Incr. group interaction. Incr. use of English language
D	F	80	CBS, paranoia, manic-depression	5.3	34	5+/1-	Incr. socially approp. behavior
E	F	90	CBS	3.6	19	1+/1-	No change
F	F	91	CBS	0.5	3 terminated	no final eval	Incr. agitation
G	F	85	CBS manic-depression	2.3	4	0+/5-	No change

INTERVENTION GROUP

68

FIGURE 3 (continued)

RESIDENT	SEX	AGE	DIAGNOSIS	YEARS IN HOME	MONTHS IN PROJECT	EVAL OUTCOME	CLINICAL OBSERVATIONS
H	F	88	CBS	3.0	24	2+/5-	Incr. confusion & suspiciousness
I	F	83	CBS hearing loss	1.1	24	1+/7-	Incr. confusion & withdrawal
J	M	82	CBS multiple CVA's	0.3	24	5+/5-	Marked incr. motor planning & social interaction
K	M	75	CBS parkinsonism	0.8	24	5+/6-	Sl. decr. participation
L	F	87	CBS rheum. arthritis	7.0	18 deceased	3+/3-	No change
M	F	86	CBS parkinsonism	4.5	10	2+/5-	Sl. decr. participation
N	F	*	R CVA (6 months)	*	8	11+/0-	Constant high level participation
O	M	91	CBS vision loss	7.0	4	7+/2-	Constant high level participation
P	M	86	CBS R CVA (7 years)	2.8	6 deceased	no final eval	Marked incr. participation. Decr. disruptive behavior

MAINTENANCE GROUP

*Information unavailable.

69

earlier) was observed to be influential in establishing trust and acceptance to the group meetings.

Olfactory stimuli presented in opening activities was observed to increase level of alertness and "tuning into" the group activities. When this was combined with interaction between residents (such as passing scented objects to one another or applying lotion in a neck rub) this was seen to increase participation for that meeting.

Inservice presentation during the course of the SP and at its conclusion were made to Jewish Home nursing and activity program staff to share the anecdotal and numerical results. This was seen to increase general staff interest in the role of sensory loss in behavior of residents with dementia and provided staff with methods to use in their interactions with residents.

Assessment results were analyzed in terms of positive and negative changes for each participant from one evaluation to the next and from initial to final assessment. Clinically, the assessment results and clinical observations determined whether a resident was or was not benefiting from participation in the project. A resident was determined to have benefited if positive changes equalled negative changes (function remained stable) or outnumbered negative changes (function improved). If assessment indicated a continued decline in function, termination from the group was considered. Upon termination, another resident was assessed for placement in the group. This happened with one group member (Resident B in Figure 3) who had become progressively more withdrawn until she was seldom interacting with SP staff or group members. At termination, she was referred for activities on a one-to-one basis when available.

Results were also used to draw some tentative conclusions about the use of the SP group format and approach in treating cognitively and sensory impaired institutionalized elderly, as well as open possible areas for further study. Several questions were asked. Were the eclectic techniques used in the SP effective in a group format for improving cognition or slowing cognitive decline? Who benefited from such a group and who did not? Was there an optimal length of time for participation? What were the factors that contributed to the success of the SP groups for those who appeared to benefit from the program?

Effectiveness of the SP Format

Based upon assessment results and clinical observations, a majority of participants (ten out of sixteen or 63%) maintained or improved cognitive and social function during their involvement in the project. Seven out of sixteen (45%) showed actual improvements in cognitive and social function. Areas of improvement most often noted included smiling, eye contact, initiation and responsiveness in conversation, and participation in group activities outside of SP meetings. While not conclusive, these results were remarkable in a population of cognitively impaired institutionalized elders.

Factors Influencing Which Residents Responded to the SP Format

Attendance. In general, those residents who attended SP meetings most regularly, benefited from them the most. However, a causal relationship cannot be assumed, since those attending most regularly may have been those most able to participate and benefit from the groups. One woman in the Maintenance Group (Resident H in Figure 3) missed many meetings near the end of the project, as she became increasingly paranoid and suspicious with the fantasy that people were trying to kill her. For a while, she seemed to trust the SP staff and to view the group meetings as a safe place. But eventually she refused more sessions as her preoccupations grew. This woman's assessment scores began declining from the beginning of her involvement in the SP groups, even before her paranoia was apparent.

Another woman who missed many group meetings during the later months of the SP was severely hearing impaired (Resident I in Figure 3). Following the group conversation may have proved too difficult for her. Even using a handheld amplification device (One-to-one Company Communicator), she missed much of the flow of the conversation, stating she felt "left out" of the discussion. This, along with ongoing lower back pain, caused her to miss many meetings. Her assessment and clinical observations data declined prior to her increasing confusion and decreasing attendance.

The third resident with poor attendance (Resident K in

Figure 3) was a man with the diagnoses of Parkinson's Disease and dementia (chronic brain syndrome); he tended to be suspicious and easily agitated. His behavior in SP meetings was significantly improved over his behavior on the nursing floor. Regardless, he was too agitated to attend SP groups after a point. While his assessment scores remained stable, his participation in meetings showed some decline in responsiveness over the two years he was a group member. In all three cases, it was impossible to determine to what degree personality and diagnosis contributed to the decline in function, which paralleled the decline in attendance.

Diagnosis. All SP participants except two had a primary diagnosis of chronic brain syndrome, with the exceptions being primary diagnoses of senile psychosis and cerebral vascular accident (CVA) with right hemiplegia, six months post. The resident with the senile psychosis was the one participant terminated during the project for consistent decline in function. The resident with the diagnosis of right hemiplegia was the member who made the most gains during the project.

Two residents with secondary diagnoses of cerebral vascular accident (one was with right hemiplegia, seven years post, and one with multiple diffuse accidents over the preceding four years) were also among the residents who improved in function during the project. Two members had secondary diagnoses of Parkinson's Disease. Both declined in function during the project. Two participants had secondary diagnoses of manic depression. One showed consistent improvement, while the other consistently declined (she was terminated for disruptiveness, as discussed above).

Group versus one-to-one treatment. Two of the residents who showed marked clinical improvement had received intensive one-to-one sensory stimulation either before or during their SP involvement. One was an 86-year-old man (Resident P in Figure 3) with the diagnosis of CVA with left hemiparesis. Nursing staff originally requested occupational therapy for this resident because his behavior had become almost unmanageable; he was throwing urinals, cursing, and constantly calling out for assistance of one sort or another. Occupational therapy evaluation revealed major deficits in perceptual skills including motor planning, spatial relations, and topographical orientation. This man did not know where he was or how to appropriately meet his basic needs. He received one-to-one sensory integration treatments including vestibular and tactile stimulation and motor planning activities three times weekly. After twelve months he was able to sit for periods up to one hour without calling for help and he began simple self care activities (upper extremity dressing and independent use of urinal). This resident then joined the Maintenance Group when an opening arose. He was in the SP program for six months. He died shortly before the project ended.

The other resident who received individual treatment was a man of 84 years with the diagnosis of multiple CVA (Resident J in Figure 3). He had been a member of the Maintenance Group from its beginning. He was observed in the group to have such severe apraxia that he was often unable to hit a balloon coming toward him or take an object being passed around the circle from the adjacent resident. He seemed acutely aware of his deficits, often choosing to abstain from activity rather than perform poorly. Outside of SP meetings he was socially withdrawn and chose to sit and stare out the window rather than attend recreation groups. One-to-one treatment was used to improve his motor planning so he could participate more easily in SP activities. After four months of three times weekly individual sensory treatment in addition to three weekly SP group meetings, this resident was able to catch and throw balls and balloons, as well as pass objects to other group members. At the conclusion of the SP, he was one of the members who has shown clinical improvement in smiling frequently, initiating conversation, attending recreation groups, and waving to staff from across the room.

Differentiating the effect of any or all of factors discussed may prove a fruitful area for further investigation. Implications for clinicians would include encouraging regular attendance and considering individual treatment when a participant is not benefiting from group treatment alone. Any conclusions about which diagnoses respond best to an eclectic sensory stimulation group treatment would be premature.

Optimal Duration of Attendance in Sensory Stimulation Groups

Of the residents who benefited from the sensory group program, three of the twelve with 2 year long data seemed to plateau in function at around 18 months of participation. Two improved until the end of the project. Periodic reassessment helped distinguish these residents. In an ongoing program, residents who have plateaued in function might best be transitioned to other types of activities.

Factors Influencing Success of SP Groups

More than half the residents who attended sensory groups maintained or improved cognitive and social function. What factors in the style or format of the meetings were influential in their success with these residents? Was it the use of sensory stimulation techniques or other factors?

Without control residents with whom to compare change in function there are no answers to these questions. The staff approach; the use of sensory stimulation activities; the group atmosphere of acceptance; the sense of community which developed among members; the consistency of time, place, and format; the opportunity to express feelings and interact with peers while engaged in sensory stimulation and sensory integration activities, which were adapted with the goal of age appropriateness, might have been more important factors or of equal significance. Meanwhile, these characteristics worked well in combination. Clinicians may experiment with group treatment of similar format and approach to offer programs for sensory and cognitively impaired institutionalized elders.

REFERENCES

Ayres, A. J. *Sensory integration and learning disorders.* Los Angeles: Western Psychological Services, 1978.

Brophy, J., Ernst, M., Shore, H. "A Short Form for Assessing Sensory Loss in the Elderly." Unpublished paper presented at 31st Annual Meeting of the Gerontological Society (Oct. 1977). Available: Center for Studies in Aging, North Texas State Univ. Denton, TX 76203.

Byron, E. M. Reversing senile behavior patterns through reality orientation-sensory group therapy. *Journal of the National Association for Private Psychiatric Hospitals,* 1978, 10, 68–72.

Carroll, K. *Compensating for Sensory Losses.* Minneapolis, MN: Ebenezer Center for Aging and Human Development, 1978.

Ebersole, P. A theoretical approach to the use of reminiscence. In I. M. Burnside (Ed.), *Working with the Elderly: Group process and techniques.* North Scituate, MA: Duxbury Press, 1978.

Feil, N. *Validation/fantasy therapy.* Cleveland, OH: Edward Feil Productions, 1980.

Fox, J. The olfactory system: Implications for the occupational therapist. *American Journal of Occupational Therapy,* 1966, 20, 173–178.

Huber, R. Sensory retraining for a fuller life. *Nursing Homes,* 1973, 22, 14–15.

Kiernat, J. M. The use of life review activity with confused nursing Home residents. *American Journal of Occupational Therapy,* 1979, 33, 306–310.

Richman, L. Sensory training for geriatric patients. *American Journal of Occupational Therapy,* 1969, 23, 254–257.

Ross, M. and D. Burdick. *Sensory integration: A training manual for therapists and teachers for regressed, psychiatric and geriatric patient groups.* New Jersey: Charles B. Slack, 1981. (The preceding edition of this reference circa 1978 was used prior to the publication of the 1981 edition.)

Wavrick, P. Sensory integration treatment with CBS patients. *Newsletter of the Center for the Study of Sensory Integration,* 1972, November, 3–4.

ASSESSMENT PROTOCOL

General Information. Diagnoses, previous occupations, special needs or precautions, and appliances used (hearing aid, eye glasses, walker or wheelchair) noted in appropriate section, after consulting the resident's medical record and nursing staff.

Activity Level. Also completed after reading the medical record and confirmed with nursing staff, this section recorded whether the resident participated in any activities on the nursing unit and which self care activities the resident accomplished independently or with assistance.

Orientation. Modified mental status questions were asked, notation was made for fully, partially or not oriented in each sphere. Time orientation was assessed by date, year, most recent holiday, resident's age, and time of day (morning, afternoon, evening). Place was assessed by inquiring about country, city, and building. Country of birth was also asked and recorded. Orientation to person was assessed by asking resident their full name, the name of their closest living relative, and the title of the person in a photograph of a nurse in uniform (as the nursing staff of Jewish Home wore traditional white uniforms). When the resident had visual deficits, the photograph was described.

Recent Memory. A stimulus of a color and a simple address were given. The resident was asked to repeat it, to ascertain that it was heard correctly. After the Sensory Perception section was filled in on the data sheet, the resident was asked to repeat the color and address.

Insight. The resident was asked, "How is your life going now?" and their response was recorded.

Body Position. Notations were made for each subsection under this heading. Head, trunk, and breathing pattern were observed at rest. Then muscle tone was assessed by both the quick stretch check to rule out the presence of spasticity and lightly palpating over muscle groups while the resident used the muscles. If the client exhibited tremors, this was noted. The resident was asked to move arms bilaterally quickly, then slowly; the quality of motion was recorded for motor planning.

Personality Characteristics. General qualities were noted here. It was recorded whether the resident was anxious, relaxed, argumentative, easy-going, cooperative or not, dependent or passive, depressed, hopeful, outgoing or quiet, self-deprecating, or self-reliant.

Range of Motion. Grossly measured without goniometer, ROM of the resident's major joints of each extremity was recorded as full or limited; if limited, this was recorded as 25%, 50%, 75% or 100% of normal range.

Strength. Recorded grossly by manual muscle test of whole muscle groups for each extremity in same manner as for range of motion.

Sensory Perception. Each subsection of perception testing was intended as a screening only. When significant deficit was found during assessment, referral to a medical specialist was made. With the data from these subtests, activities were adapted during group meetings to facilitate participation and to develop an accurate understanding of each group member's functional status. The results of this portion of the assessment were shared with nursing staff.

Vision. Near vision was assessed by asking the resident to read a standardized Berens card available at optical supply companies for use by optometrists and ophthamologists. Reading glasses were worn for this. Distance vision was assessed grossly by holding the standard Snellen Eye Chart at a five foot distance from the resident and having them read as far down as possible. For distractible individuals, this was modified by folding the chart into sections of two and one half inches and revealing only one section at a time.

Audition. Perception of high and low frequency sounds were assessed by playing a tape player with four sentences repeated four times each at increasing volume to determine functionally what each resident heard best. A tape of a woman making a statement with varying background sounds was used to similarly determine whether the resident would be able to participate in group meetings when extraneous sounds were present and was recorded on the auditory figure ground line of the sheet. This also indicated a resident's frustration tolerance and irritability level. Notations were made on the data sheet when these pieces of information surfaced.

Proprioception. This was assessed in the usual manner in rehabilitation settings.

Sterognosis. As above.

Taste. The resident was given five stimulus cups, each containing a different tasting liquid and covered by an opaque lid; water was in one cup as a validity control. The resident was asked to determine whether any flavor was detected, and if so, what flavor was detected. Between each stimulus cup, water was used to rinse the mouth.

Olfaction. Three fragrances were presented and the response (identifying the type of scent) was recorded. Vials were covered and one was empty for control.

Visual Pursuits. Three motions of a pencil were followed by the resident; whether or not it was followed fully and whether or not the resident's eyes crossed midline without jerking were noted.

Auditory Memory. The numbers on the form were said slowly and the resident was asked to repeat. How many digits were repeated correctly was written as the score.

Equilibrium. If the resident could stand, the Romberg test was given with eyes open and closed if tolerated.

Trunk Rotation. While twisting to each side once, the resident was observed for whether or not resident could reach an object held at 65 degrees to the side to which they turned. This provided information about ability of resident to motor plan and work in a gravity eliminated position.

Integration of Reflexes. Evaluated in sitting with arms at 60 degrees of shoulder forward flexion. Resident was asked to look toward right, then left, then up and then down. Ability to move head without producing muscle tone change in arms was recorded, as was presence of tactile defensiveness.

Body Awareness. How long it took resident to correctly respond to the instruction was recorded, as was accuracy.

Intersensory Graphesthesia. Ability to follow directions and tolerance of the evaluator's finger drawing the letter on the palm of one hand was recorded. Accuracy for identifying the letter was noted.

Imitation of Postures. Ability to copy exactly what the evaluator does is recorded. Attention was given to moving swiftly to avoid giving motor planning cues, the time was measured by counting until resident completed posture and accuracy was recorded by circling description.

Ability to Follow Directions. General ability as seen throughout all tasks is noted.

Attention Span/Level of Alertness. Notations were made based on performance during the full assessment.

APPENDIX

Jewish Home for the Aged
Sensory Awareness Training Project
Assessment Data Sheet

Name   Date

General Information
      Diagnosis
      Occupation(s)
      Precautions
      Appliances

Activity Level
      Type, Frequency of Activities
      Amount of Self Care

Orientation
      Time
      Place
      Person

Recent Memory

Insight

Body Position/ Motor Planning
      Head
      Trunk
      Breathing Pattern, Direction of Gaze
      Muscle Tone
      Body Parts in Motion
      Motor Planning

Personality Characteristics

Range of Motion R U/E   L U/E
                    R L/E   L L/E
Strength R U/E   L U/E
                R L/E   L L/E

Sensory Perception
      Vision Near   Distance
      Audition Frequency, High   Low
                    Volume   Figure Ground
      Proprioception
            R U/E
            L U/E
      Stereognosis Right   Left
      Taste
            Discrimination Salty/Bitter/Control/Sweet/Sour
            Identification Salty/Bitter/Control/Sweet/Sour

Olfaction
    Discrimination Flower-Fruit/Control/Musky/Putrid
    Identification Flower-Fruit/Control/Musky/Putrid

Visual Pursuits
  Smooth   Quick   Convergence

Auditory Memory   Score
  713   2836   42596

Equilibrium
    Romberg Eyes Open
             Eyes Closed
    Modified Eyes Open
           Eyes Closed

Trunk Rotation
    Sitting Right   Left
    Standing Right   Left

Integration of Reflexes
    ATNR Rotation of neck to Right
    ATNR Rotation of neck to Left
    STNR Neck Flexion
    STNR Neck Extension
    Tactile Defensiveness Noted

Body Awareness
    Show me your right hand   sec.
    Touch your nose   sec.
    Touch your left ear   sec.
    Touch your right knee   sec.
    Show me your left foot   sec.

Intersensory Graphesthesia
      directions   defensiveness
    T   sec.   Repeat   Errors
    S   sec.   Repeat   Errors
    B   sec.   Repeat   Errors

Imitation of Postures
    Hands on Face-Cross Midline   sec. Accur. Near Inacc.
    Bend, Hands to Ear   sec. Accur. Near Inacc.
    Hands, Knee & Cheek-Cross Midline sec. Accur. Near Inacc.

Ability to Follow Instructions
Attention Span/Level of Alertness
Comments

Acknowlegements: Ayres, 1978
                   Brophy, 1977
                   Ross and Burdick, 1981

The Occupational Therapist's Role in Geropsychiatry Interdisciplinary Team Evaluation

Frances A. Kelley, OTR

ABSTRACT. The purpose of this report is to describe the development and function of an outpatient geropsychiatry evaluation clinic at Sepulveda Veterans Administration Medical Center. The team structure, evaluation instrument and processes are described with emphasis on the occupational therapist's use of Pfeiffer's Fundamental Assessment Inventory segment on Physical and Instrumental Activities of Daily Living and Matsutsusyu's Neuropsychiatric Institute Interest Check List. The occupational therapist on the outpatient geropsychiatry evaluation team assesses function and interest in vocational, avocational and daily living activities.

DEVELOPMENT OF THE GEROPSYCHIATRY EVALUATION CLINIC

The Veterans Administration Medical Center at Sepulveda, California is actively concerned with the identification, remedy and prevention of the problems of the elderly veteran. Being one of ten settings in the nation for a Geriatric Research Education and Clinical Center (GRECC) has resulted in many studies and programs including a Fellowship in Geri-

---

Frances A. Kelley, Chief, Occupational Therapy, VAMC (117D), 16111 Plummer, Sepulveda, CA 91343.

Acknowledgments: Veterans Administration Medical Center, Sepulveda, CA; Adelita D. Bonebakker, M. D., Chief Rehabilitation Medicine Service; Jaime Fitten, M.D., Chief Geropsychiatry Service; Toni Kawamoto, O.T.R., Clinical Education Specialist; Madelyne Johnston, Occupational Therapy Volunteer, Emily Stabelfeldt, manuscript preparation.

81

atric Medicine, a Geriatric Evaluation Unit (GEU) and Inter-disciplinary Team Training in Geriatrics (ITTG).

GRECC also works closely with the recently developed Geropsychiatry Service. The Chief of this Service, L. Jaime Fitten, M.D., has specialties in Psychiatry and Internal Medicine and subspecialty training in Geriatric Medicine. He established the Geropsychiatry Outpatient Clinic at VAMC, Sepulveda, about two years ago. Through his fellowship in Geriatric Medicine (Gero Med), it became obvious to Dr. Fitten that there were a large number of patients with cognitive and emotional impairments needing psychological/psychiatric evaluation not available in the Gero-Med Program and that a more comprehensive approach to diagnosis and treatment was needed. To be effective, however, geropsychiatry evaluation could not stop with behavioral manifestations of cognitive or affective limitation in the elderly, but needed to include assessment of medical problems and psychosocial variations as well as individual functional ability (Kane, 1981). To accomplish this required the interdisciplinary team approach. Dr. Fitten brought together a large base of professionals capable of providing a variety of needed interventions: medical, psychological, social and functional. Thus organized the Gero-Psychiatry Out Patient Clinic became an important entry point for elderly patients needing psychiatric and psychosocial intervention (Fitten, 1985).

Clinic's Functions

The Geropsychiatry Out Patient Clinic not only evaluates, but provides consultant services and serves as a treatment clinic. After a comprehensive evaluation, the interdisciplinary team (IT) determines more specific evaluations, social and/or therapeutic interventions. The same battery of data is collected on all patients for comparison, study and evaluation of the team's own interventions.

The team's initial evaluation may indicate a need for more specialized consultation, i.e., referral to the Cerebral Dysfunction Clinic, Geropsychiatry In-Patient Unit, Rehabilitation Medicine Service or other medical center services. Treatment offered by the clinic provides psychosocial interventions, psychotherapy (group and individual), Alzheimer's support group for significant others, pharmacotherapy, home evaluations, referrals to existing medical center programs for supportive and/or remedial interventions, and additional evaluation.

All patients are also evaluated in Gero Med where stronger emphasis is on medical problems and physical limitations. Through referrals from either Gero Med or Gero Psychiatry Services, patients may be seen by a physiatrist and appropriately referred to Occupational Therapy, Physical Therapy, or Corrective Therapy which may include driver assessment and training.

Clinic Structure and Process

Clinic patients are referred from the hospital at large, the Gero Med Service and other geriatric services. The clinic meets once a week for four hours. Three hours are devoted to interviewing, data collection and individual and group therapies. During the last hour the team meets to discuss patients whose evaluations have been completed. The team is composed of professionals who are interested in geropsychiatry and can provide time to the program. Certain staff members are hired specifically for the program and trainees from several disciplines also participate. The interdisciplinary team includes the occupational therapist, the geropsychiatrist, psychologist, nurse, social worker, pharmacist, social science research specialist/group therapist and the program coordinator.

Evaluation instruments used by team members are segments of the Functional Assessment Inventory (FAI) developed by Eric Pfeiffer, M.D. (Pfeiffer, 1982) and Part I of the Neuropsychiatric Institute Interest Check List (NPI ICL) created by Janice S. Matsutsuyu, M.A., O.T.R. (Matsusuyu, 1969). The FAI has four segments: (1) Physical and Instrumental Activities of Daily Living (ADL & IADL), (2) Sociodemographic, (3) Physical Health and, (4) Short Portable Mental Status Questionnaire (SPMSQ). Each segment has a rating scale and questions for interviewer impressions. The segments are done by four different team members. Part I of the NPI ICL is a check list of 80 activities, has a scoring sheet and is done by the occupational therapist.

Members of the team administer the different segments and all of the data collected on an individual patient is shared and corroborated during the team meeting. The team meeting is facilitated by the clinic coordinator and two to three patients can be discussed in the hour meeting. The interdisciplinary team members report their findings based on the evaluations utilized and a discussion is generated to identify problems, consider possible diagnosis, make recommendations, referrals and finally a comprehensive treatment plan for each patient.

Occupational Therapy Role

The occupational therapist's evaluation is titled Vocational/ Avocational and is composed of the ADL and IADL segment of the FAI, Part 1 of the NPI ICL and introductory questions asking (1) highlights of work experience and (2) activities being done for fun/pleasure. The evaluation material and rating information are contained in the Appendix. The process is self-report by the person being evaluated and/or significant other (if present) and usually takes about 20 to 30 minutes. The O.T. evaluation focus is on function and the objectives are to identify how the person occupies himself, the activities he does and does not do, his interests and attitudes in relation to activities, what can be done to improve his functional ability and quality of life. Interpretation of this data in conjunction with data shared by the team has contributed significantly by pointing out (1) limitations in ADL and IADL function that are indicative of memory problems or depression and (2) interest patterns that are related to moods, remembering, problem solving, decision making and quality of life experiences (Mace, 1981).

Seven IADL activities and eight ADL activities (fifteen in the entire segment) are addressed by the FAI Physical and Instrumental ADL segment (see Appendix A, B). Each activity is rated on a three level scale of the person's ability to do the activity without any help, with some help or unable to do it at all. Performance is rated on a six-point scale from excellent ADL capacity to completely impaired ADL capacity (see Appendix C). Additional information about the interview and the subject are obtained by 6 questions answered by the interviewer (see Appendix D). All of the IADL and the second, third, sixth and eighth activities of the ADL involve cognitive as well as physical function. Indications of dysfunction may be quite obvious if severe or very subtle if mild. Some repeatedly seen responses to the fifteen activities indicative of memory problems validated by team discussion are as follows: (1) not using the telephone because "don't know what to say," "can't" or other responses not related to ability to hear or physically manage the telephone, (2) always goes places with another person; may wait in the car during shopping trips when there is no problem with ambulation or endurance, (3) is not reading or writing, i.e., taking messages, writing checks, (4) someone else manages the medication, (5) needs help shaving or gets help shaving or gets help shaving because the helper isn't satisfied with the way he does it, (7) needs help bathing, i.e., adjusting the water temperature, (8) problem getting to the bathroom on time.

Team discussion plays an important and necessary part in determining the core problems, rehab potential, possibility of improving quality of life and/or whether additional evaluation is needed.

The NPI ICL gives information about the expressed interest of the person being evaluated (see Appendix E). The data is systematized into the five categories of Manual Skill, Social Recreation, Cultural/Educational and ADL. The three expressions of strength of interest are Casual, Strong and NO (see Appendix F). The check list was created so that the occupational therapist would have a systematic collection of data to provide valid information from which to build an environment that would set standards for skilled instruction and protect a patient's right to hope and to learn (Matsutsuyu, 1969). In the geropsychiatry clinic evaluation process the ICL provides interest patterns that can suggest problems related to moods, remembering, problem solving and decision making. Some significant responses and behaviors have been: (1) person being evaluated having trouble understanding that desired response is *interest* rather than *participation,* (2) contradictory information with other elements of evaluation i.e., activities stated as those done for pleasure are rated "no" interest on the ICL, (3) remarks revealing that the person remembers that he does forget, (4) ability to read, comprehend and make choices will be demonstrated if the person does the ICL independently, (5) focus on past or "used to do" interests and being vague about recent interests, (6) strong interests can be identified as activities done alone or activities done with others, (7) large numbers of "casual" responses (suggest indecisiveness), (8) large number of "no" responses (suggest denial).

Information and discussion shared with other team members to give more of the total picture makes the meaning of these responses and behaviors more obvious.

The introductory questions about work/experience and fun/pleasure are asked first and are kept brief. Their purpose, in addition to the information gained, is to focus the person's thinking on the positive aspects of daily living, past and present, and to emphasize his capabilities rather than limitations.

The occupational therapist's evaluation is less intrusive and less threatening than other segments of the evaluation and tends to bring out positive interests and experiences. Identifying the person's own reference of quality experience has been useful to the team in assessing potential motivation and response to proposed treatment.

CONCLUSION

The value of the team structure and approach is essential. The findings of different evaluators validate each other and the variety of evaluation foci makes subtle dysfunctions more apparent.

Evaluation tends to stimulate research activity (Fozard, 1985). Some occupational therapy research needs have become apparent from this program: (1) follow-up assessments regarding accuracy of initial assessments and effectiveness of treatment plans, (2) evaluation as an instrument to measure positive or negative indications of quality of life, (3) the influence and importance of senior/day centre psychosocial encounters, (4) the value of cognitive rehabilitation through structured, purposeful activities, (5) benefits of home evaluations, i.e., determining spouse's needs, safety in the home, utilization of work simplification techniques, (6) the need for training in meal preparation and planning.

REFERENCES

Fitten, Jaime. Interview. Sepulveda V.A. Medical Center, 1985.
Kane, Rosalie A., & Kane, Robert L. *Assessing the elderly.* Lexington. Lexington Books, 1981.
Mace, Nancy L. & Rabins, Peter V. *The 36-hour day.* Baltimore. The Johns Hopkins University Press, 1981.
Matsutsuyu, Janice S. The interest check list. *American Journal of Occupational Therapy,* 1969, *23,* 323-328.
Pfeiffer, Eric. Functional assessment inventory. University of South Florida, 1982.
Fozard, James, Ph.D. Comprehensive Geriatric Evaluation In the V.A. and the Role Behavioral Scientists Play. *Geriatric Grand Rounds.* V.A.M.C., Sepulveda, 1985.

BIBLIOGRAPHY

Beaver, Marion L. *Human Service With the Elderly.* Prentice-Hall, Inc. Englewood Cliffs, New Jersey 07632. 1983.
Brink, T. L., & Yesavage, Jerome A. Screening Tests for Geriatric Depression. *Clinical Gerontologist.* Vol. 1, 1, Fall 1982, 37.
Gregory, Mark D. Occupational Behavior & Life Satisfaction Among Retirees. (meaningful activities, retirement, adaptation) *American Journal of Occupational Therapy,* 1983, 548.
National Institutes of Health. (Revised Aug. 1980) *Guide to Medical Self-care and Self-help Groups for the Elderly.* (NIH Publication No. 80-1687.) Washington, D.C.
Gummow, Linda J. PhD, Macnamar, Susan, Dustman, Robert E., PhD, Cognitive Rehabilitation and the Elderly Veteran. *VA Practitioner.* Vol. 2, Number 2, Feb. 1985. VAMC, Salt Lake City, Utah.
Kaplan, Jerome. Evaluation Techniques for Older Groups. *American Journal of Occupational Therapy.* 1959, Vol. 13, 5.
Maurer, Patti, PhD, OTR, Barris, Roamon, EdD, OTR, Bouder, Betty, PhD, OTR, & Gillett, Nedra, MEd, OTR. Hierarchy of Competencies Relating to the Use Of Standardized Instruments and Evaluation Techniques by Occupational Therapists. *American Journal of Occupational Therapy.* December 1985, 38, 12.
National Advisory Council on Aging. (January 1980). *Our Future Selves.* Report of the Panel on Behavioral and Social Sciences Research. (NIH Publication. 80-1444), Washington, DC.
Pfeiffer, Eric, MD, Functional Assessment Inventory. University of South Florida College of Medicine, Tampa, Florida, 1982.
Pincus, Allen, PhD. New Findings on Learning in Old Age—Implications for Occupational Therapy. *American Journal of Occupational Therapy.* 1968, 22, 4.
Principles of Occupational Therapy Ethics. Rockville, MD. The American Occupational Therapy Association, Inc., adopted, revised, April 1979.
Schaffer, Charles B., MD and Donlon, Patrick T., MD. Medical Causes of Psychiatric Symptoms in the Elderly. *Clinical Gerontologist.* Summer 1983, 1, 4.
Standards of Practice for Occupational Therapy. Rockville, MD. The American Occupational Therapy Association, Inc. Adapted by the Representative Assembly. April 1983.
Strauss, Donald, MSW, and Soloman, Keneth, MD. Psychopharmacologic Intervention for Depression in the Elderly. *Clinical Gerontologist.* Summer 1983, 1, 4.

Tickle, Linda S., & Yerxa, Elizabeth J. Need Satisfaction of Older Persons Living in the Community and in Institutions, Part 2, Role of Activity. *American Journal of Occupational Therapy,* Oct. 1981, 650.

Winston, Ellen B. An Older Population: Meeting Major Needs Through Occupational Therapy. *American Journal of Occupational Therapy,* Oct. 1981, 635, 645, 650.

APPENDIX A

Activities of Daily Living

Now I'd like to ask you about some of the activities of daily living, things that we all need to do as part of our daily lives. I would like to know if you can do these activities without any help at all, or if you need some help to do them, or if you can't do them at all. (BE SURE TO READ ALL ANSWER CHOICES IF APPLICABLE IN QUESTIONS 53 THROUGH 68.)

Instrumental ADL

53. Can you use the telephone . . .

    1 without help, including looking up numbers and dialing
    2 with some help (can answer phone or dial operator in an emergency but need a special phone or help in getting the number or dialing)
    3 or are you completely unable to use the telephone?

54. Can you get to places out of walking distance . . .

    1 without help (can travel alone on buses, taxis, or drive your own car)
    2 with some help (need someone to help you or go with you when traveling)
    3 or are you unable to travel unless emergency arrangements are made for a specialized vehicle like an ambulance?

55. Can you go shopping for groceries or clothes (ASSUMING PERSON HAS TRANSPORTATION) . . .

    1 without help (taking care of all shopping needs yourself, assuming you had transportation)
    2 with some help (need someone to go with you on all shopping trips)
    3 or are you completely unable to do any shopping?

56. Can you prepare your own meals . . .

    1 without help (plan and cook full meals yourself)
    2 with some help (can prepare some things but unable to cook full meals yourself)
    3 or are you completely unable to prepare any meals?
57. Can you do your housework . . .

    1 without help (can scrub floors, etc.)
    2 with some help (can do light housework but need help with heavy work)
    3 or are you completely unable to do any housework?
58. Can you take your own medicine . . .

    1 without help (in the right doses and at the right times)
    2 with some help (able to take medicine if someone prepares it for you and/or reminds you to take it)
    3 or are you completely unable to take your medicines?
59. Can you handle you own money . . .

    1 without help (write checks, pay bills, etc.)
    2 with some help (manage day-to-day buying but need help with managing your checkbook and paying your bills)
    3 or are you completely unable to handle money?

APPENDIX B

Physical ADL

60. Can you eat . . .

    1 without help (able to feed yourself completely)
    2 with some help (need help with cutting, etc.)
    3 or are you completely unable to feed yourself?
61. Can you dress and undress yourself . . .

    1 without help (able to pick out clothes, dress and undress yourself)
    2 with some help
    3 or are you completely unable to dress and undress yourself?

62. Can you take care of your own appearance, for example combing your hair and (for men) shaving . . .

    1 without help
    2 with some help
    3 or are you completely unable to maintain your appearance yourself?

63. Can you walk . . .

    1 without help (except from a cane)
    2 with some help from a person (or with the use of a walker, or crutches, etc.)
    3 or are you completely unable to walk?

64. Can you get in and out of bed . . .

    1 without any help or aids
    2 with some help (either from a person or with the aid of some device)
    3 or are you totally dependent on someone else to lift you?

65. Can you take a bath or shower . . .

    1 without help
    2 with some help (need help getting in and out of the tub, or need special attachments on the tub)
    3 or are you completely unable to bathe yourself?

66. Do you ever have trouble getting to the bathroom on time?

    1 No
    2 Occasionally
    3 Frequently

67. During the past six months have you had any help with such things as shopping, housework, bathing, dressing, and getting around?

    1 Yes
    2 No

(IF "YES" ASK 68.)

68. Who is your major helper? (SPECIFY) Name: _____
    Relationship: 1. husband or wife
                  2. other relative
                  3. friend

APPENDIX C

Performance Rating Scale for Activities of Daily Living

94. (RATE THE CURRENT PERFORMANCE OF THE PERSON BEING EVALUATED ON THE SIX-POINT SCALE PRESENTED BELOW. CIRCLE THE *ONE* NUMBER WHICH BEST DESCRIBES THE PERSON'S PRESENT PERFORMANCE. ACTIVITIES OF DAILY LIVING QUESTIONS ARE NUMBERS 53–68.)

1. *Excellent ADL capacity.*
   Can perform all of the Activities of Daily Living without assistance and with ease.
2. *Good ADL capacity.*
   Can perform all of the Activities of Daily Living without assistance.
3. *Mildly impaired ADL capacity.*
   Can perform all but one to three of the Activities of Daily Living. Some help is required with one to three, but not necessarily every day. Can get through any single day without help. Is able to prepare his own meals.
4. *Moderately impaired ADL capacity.*
   Regularly requires assistance with at least four Activities of Daily Living but is able to get through any single day without help. Or regularly requires help with meal preparation.
5. *Severely impaired ADL capacity.*
   Need help each day but not necessarily throughout the day or night with many of the Activities of Daily Living.
6. *Completely impaired ADL capacity.*
   Needs help throughout the day and/or night to carry out the Activities of Daily Living.

APPENDIX D

(THE REMAINING QUESTIONS ARE TO BE ANSWERED BY THE INTERVIEWER IMMEDIATELY
AFTER COMPLETING THE INTERVIEW.)

84. Length of interview _____
                                              (Minutes

85. Factual information obtained from:
    1 Subject
    2 Relative
    3 Other (SPECIFY) _____

86. Factual questions (obtained from Subject and/or informant) are:
    1 Completely reliable
    2 Reliable on most items
    3 Reliable on only a few items
    4 Completely unreliable

87. Subjective questions (those in boxes, obtained from Subject only) are:
    1 Completely reliable
    2 Reliable on most items
    3 Reliable on only a few items
    4 Completely unreliable
    5 Not obtained

    (IF 5 ANSWER 88.)

88. Why didn't the Subject answer the Subjective questions? (BE SPECIFIC)

    _____

    _____

    _____

    _____

89. During the interview did the Subject's behavior strike you as:
    (CIRCLE "YES" OR "NO" FOR EACH OF THE FOLLOWING.)

            1   2

a.   YES no   Mentally alert and stimulating
b.   YES no   Pleasant and cooperative
c.   YES no   Depressed and/or tearful
d.   YES no   Withdrawn or lethargic
e.   YES no   Fearful, anxious or extremely tense
f.   YES no   Full of unrealistic physical complaints
g.   YES no   Suspicious (more than reasonable)
h.   YES no   Bizarre or inappropriate in thought or action
i.   YES no   Excessively talkative or overly jovial or elated

APPENDIX E

Interest Check List *
_____
Assessment Instrument

Date:_____

Subject:_____

Examiner:_____

*Please check each item below according to your interest.

ACTIVITY	Casual	Strong	No	ACTIVITY	Casual	Strong	No
1.Gardening				41.Exercise			
2.Sewing				42.Volleyball			
3.Poker				43.Woodworking			
4.Languages				44.Billiards			
5.Social Clubs				45.Driving			
6.Radio				46.Dusting			
7.Bridge				47.Jewelry Making			
8.Car Repair				48.Tennis			
9.Writing				49.Cooking			
10.Dancing				50.Basketball			
11.Needlework				51.History			
12.Golf				52.Guitar			
13.Football				53.Science			
14.Popular Music				54.Collecting			
15.Puzzles				55.Ping Pong			
16.Holidays				56.Leatherwork			
17.Solitaire				57.Shopping			
18.Movies				58.Photography			
19.Lectures				59.Painting			
20.Swimming				60.Television			
21.Bowling				61.Concerts			
22.Visiting				62.Ceramics			
23.Mending				63.Camping			
24.Chess				64.Laundry			
25.Barbecues				65.Dating			
26.Reading				66.Mosaics			
27.Traveling				67.Politics			
28.Manual Arts				68.Scrabble			
29.Parties				69.Decorating			
30.Dramatics				70.Math			
31.Shuffleboard				71.Service Groups			
32.Ironing				72.Piano			
33.Social Studies				73.Scouting			
34.Classical Music				74.Plays			
35.Floor Mopping				75.Clothes			
36.Model Building				76.Knitting			
37.Baseball				77.Hairstyling			
38.Checkers				78.Religion			
39.Singing				79.Drums			
40.Home Repairs				80.Conversation			

*Please list other special interests:

APPENDIX F

Items:

Manual	Soc.Rec.		Cult.Ed.	Phys. Spt.	ADL
CSN	CSN		CSN	CSN	
1.	3.	4.	12.		23.
2.	5.	9.	13.		32.
8.	6.	19.	20.		35.
11.	7.	26.	21.		40.
28.	10.	27.	31.		45.
36.	14.	30.	37.		46.
43.	15.	33.	41.		49.
47.	16.	34.	42.		57.
56.	17.	51.	48.		64.
62.	18.	52.	50.		75.
66.	22.	53.	55.		
76.	24.	54.			
77.	25.	58.			
	29.	59.			
	38.	61.			
	39.	67.			
	44.	69.			
	60.	70.			
	63.	72.			
	65.	74.			
	68.	78.			
	71.	79.			
	73.				
	80.				

Number of Responses:

Strong	Strong	Strong	Strong	Strong
Casual	Casual	Casual	Casual	Casual
No	No	No	No	No

Inferences and Summary

Day Care and Alzheimer's Disease: A Weekend Program in New York City

Ellen Rabinowitz, OTR

ABSTRACT. Relatively few day care programs have been established exclusively for individuals with Alzheimer's Disease. Of the limited number of such programs in the New York City area, there is currently only one that operates on Saturday. The Day Activities Program at the New York Institute for Aging is staffed entirely by occupational therapy personnel.

A description of the program follows including intake procedure, clinical characteristics of participants, physical environment, staffing patterns, and activities that have been found to be successful with mild to moderately demented individuals.

INTRODUCTION

It is estimated that four to five percent of the over-65 population have severe dementia and 11–12 percent have mild to moderate dementia. This translates into more than three million people.[1] The most common form of dementia is Alzheimer's Disease, and most Alzheimer's victims are cared for by their families at home.[2] Only a small percentage of Alzheimer's victims in the community are using day care services. This is due in part to the fact that very few adult day centers in the United States service Alzheimer's patients.[3] In the New York City area, there are fewer than five day programs geared *exclusively* to the unique needs of patients with de-

---

Ellen Rabinowitz holds a Bachelor of Science degree in Occupational Therapy and is completing a Master's Degree in Gerontology. She is in private practice and is Coordinator of the Day Activities Program at the New York Institute for Aging, 119 East 36th Street, New York, NY 10016.

95

mentia. Following is a description of one such program, the Day Activities Program at the New York Institute for Aging (NYIA).

The Institute is a private facility devoted solely to the care of geriatric patients and their families. The NYIA staff is multi-disciplinary, and includes a psychiatrist, psychologists, social workers, a psychiatric nurse, gerontologists, and since the inception of the day program, occupational therapists. The majority of the Institute's clients have been diagnosed as having Alzheimer's disease or a related dementia. A smaller number of clients suffer from depression and other affective disorders. The NYIA offers a wide range of services including diagnostic evaluation, psychological testing, pharmacological treatment for symptom management, medical supervision, in-home visits and case management, family support groups, legal and financial counseling and referral, and most recently, a day program. The Day Program was initiated in December, 1984.

THE NYIA DAY PROGRAM

The Day Activities Program (DAP) at the New York Institute for Aging is a Saturday only program. Saturday was chosen for two reasons: first, other dementia day programs in New York City operated on weekdays only, and second, many caregivers have full or part-time help during the week, but are alone with the Alzheimer's victim on the weekend. The NYIA Alzheimer's day program is still the only such weekend program in New York City.

The DAP is designed specifically for patients with memory and cognitive impairments. Our purpose is two-fold: to provide a variety of stimulating activities for participants, and to offer much needed weekend respite for their caregivers. The program operates from 10 A.M. to 3 P.M. each Saturday. The participant's family is responsible for transporting the participant to and from the program. Participants are usually accompanied by a home health aide or family member. Only two clients have been able to travel to the center independently.

Each participant's family is also responsible for the cost of the program. There is a fixed, per-day fee of $50 for the DAP. This fee is consistent with that of other programs in the

New York metropolitan area, but would vary in other parts of the country based upon the actual costs of running such a program (including staff salaries, food and other supplies for group activities, and overhead expenses such as rent).

Due to space limitations (physical layout described elsewhere) the maximum number of participants the DAP can accommodate is twelve. Our current census is eight, four of whom have been in the program since its inception. Presently, participants range in age from 59 to 87, and are equally divided by sex. Regular participation in the program is encouraged, however, a small number of participants attend the program on alternate Saturdays only.

Admission to the program is based on an interview with the participant and his caregiver, as well as a written application completed by the caregiver. The interview is conducted by a psychologist and a registered occupational therapist. The written application contains pertinent medical information, an interest checklist, and the caregiver's report of the client's ADL abilities. In addition, the application asks about allergies to foods or animals (cooking and pet therapy are integral activities in the program). Following two weeks in the program, an occupational therapy assessment is completed on each participant.

Restricted from the DAP are participants who are wheelchair-bound, incontinent, or too agitated to sustain group participation. Unfortunately, the physical premises are not wheelchair accessible, nor is there ample space in the bathroom for a staff member to change an incontinent client. Frequent reminders (every two hours) as to location of the bathroom are offered, and participants are encouraged to use bathroom facilities after lunch. In terms of behavioral problems, only one person has been discharged from the program due to severe agitation; this was following four weeks of participation during which time she was unable to be calmed by staff, family members, or a clinical trial of medication. The most common reason for discharge from the DAP is transfer to a higher level of care (nursing home). Less frequent reasons for withdrawal from the program are cost and travel limitations.

Participants in the DAP can be clinically characterized as stage four (Late Confusional/Mild Alzheimer's disease) or stage five (Early Dementia/Moderate Alzheimer's Disease) of Reisberg's Global Deterioration Scale.[4] Common characteristics of these stages and the DAP participants include impaired concentration and attention span, decreased awareness of current events, disorientation to time, place or season, inability to recall address and/or telephone number, inability to travel independently, and some difficulty recalling names of siblings or grandchildren. Invariably, day program participants know their own names, and the name of the spouse, child, or aide who constantly cares for them. Consistent with Reisberg's stages four and five, on a functional level participants are unable to handle finances and marketing, and may have difficulty choosing clothing that is appropriate.

PHYSICAL LAYOUT

The NYIA is located in an urban area, on the East side of Manhattan, in New York City. The Institute has space in a recently refurbished townhouse building, on the garden level (one floor below the street level entrance). The garden level is accessible by stairs or a small elevator. The space occupied by the NYIA consists of a small office that is approximately twelve feet by twelve feet and has a sliding glass door that opens onto a small enclosed concrete patio. Connecting the two offices is a long hallway which houses the elevator, stairway, bathroom, and kitchen area. The kitchen is a closet, about three feet wide by four feet deep, but contains a refrigerator, sink, and range top with two burners. Well-placed shelving allows for storage of food, pots and pans, and other utensils. This area was constructed specifically for the day program.

A number of environmental modifications take place every Saturday morning to make the atmosphere less "office-like" and more beneficial for the functioning of the DAP participants. Signs are posted identifying the elevator door, bathroom, and meeting room (the larger office). Participant artwork is placed (temporarily) in the meeting room and hallway. In addition, a sign is placed under the clock in the hallway, which reads "Everyone goes home at 3:00." The small office is used for storage of participants' coats and handbags. Each personal item a participant leaves in the small room is affixed with a spring-type clothespin which has the participant's name on it. The door to this room is then closed, so that coats are out of sight. This room is also used on occasions when a client required one to one attention for a limited period of time.

In the hallway, a small table is placed in front of the stairs as a safety precaution, and the elevator sign is turned over and the elevator light is turned off. Our goal is to keep participants from wandering off, yet allow them to move about in the hallway if they need to do so. No participant has ever wandered out of the building undetected, though on a few occasions a participant has been escorted on a walk around the block to shed excess energy.

The larger room is used for most of our groups. A reality orientation board is hung up and there are a calendar and clock readily available for orientation purposes. We have found that participants are more relaxed when the drapes are pulled back and they are afforded a view of the outside. This again helps with orientation, as we are able to see snow, rain, sunshine and leaves changing color as the seasons pass. A final assistive device is that all participants and staff wear name tags, with first names printed clearly in a dark color on a white background. If the group leaves the building for an outing, however, name tags are dispensed with to avoid participant's feelings of self-consciousness.

STAFFING

The staff to participant ratio in the DAP is one to three. Depending on the number of participants on a given day, the program is staffed by one registerd occupational therapist and one or two occupational therapy students. Students are re- cruited from Bachelor's and Master's-level occupational ther- apy programs in the New York City area, and are trained and informally supervised by the registered occupational therap- ists on an ongoing basis. The students are paid a small stipend for their work; they are part-time employees of the NYIA and their work at the DAP does not take the place of clinical affiliations.

All staff work together planning activities, co-leading groups, and giving feedback to family members. The current staff for the day program consists of two registered occupational therapists and four occupational therapy students; all staff is rotated in "round-robin" fashion so that each OTR has the opportunity to work with each student. Staff meetings are held at least once every three months to keep abreast of scheduling problems and pertinent patient issues.

Since occupational therapists are the only staff present during the DAP, the Institute's psychiatrist is available "on-call" should medical or pharmacological issues arise, and a social worker is available "on-call" should a complex family issue arise that demands immediate attention.

TYPICAL ACTIVITIES

The occupational therapy staff is responsible for planning the program's activities on a week-to-week basis. A variety of therapeutic activities are utilized, and we have found that activities of short duration (30–45 minutes) are most successful, with plenty of time between groups for coffee breaks or a simple stretch. Groups are set up in a circle or around a table, to promote cohesion.

A typical day begins with basic reality orientation: location, date, weather and next holiday. A review is made of the names of all who are present, as well as reminders such as a participant who has medication to take at a certain time during the course of the day. While basic reality orientation information is available for reference, it is not stressed, as dementia patients have no recollection of current events and have little or no recall memory. Rather, participants are led into a reminiscence group focusing on holiday traditions, neighborhoods, or countries of origin. An attempt is made to find a common interest or bond between participants and discuss past events, which remain more clearly intact in an Alzheimer's victim's memory. This verbal group is usually followed by a movement and music group.

Exercises that utilize concrete objects seem to be easier for the participants to follow than exercises requiring just movement of body parts. For example, an elastic jumprope, held by all participants, may be stretched forward and backward, up and down, and side to side. Twelve-inch long wooden dowels are used to stimulate movements such as stirring soup, rowing a boat, leading an orchestra, or hitting a baseball. The participant who is confused seems better able to exercise with an object, and following the imitative directions of the group leader. Our participants particularly enjoy the balloon toss, which increases eye-hand coordination, cooperation, and allows them to enjoy themselves and laugh. At times we will also kick around a beach ball for lower extremity movement, but this tends to get participants very excited and it seems more difficult for them to direct their energy. Older participants become afraid of this activity at times, whereas the balloon is less threatening. Throughout the exercise session, familiar music is played, with varying tempos to suit the mood of the group.

An integral part of the DAP is meal preparation. Cooking seems to be a skill that is retained even in moderately confused individuals, and is practical because participants can assist caregivers with meal preparation at home. One of the DAP clients and one of the occupational therapy students shop for the ingredients necessary for the day's lunch. A typical meal might be soup, chef's salad, buttered rolls, instant pudding and beverage, or sandwiches, macaroni and cheese, fruit salad and beverage. We attempt to have a balanced meal that requires much preparation in the form of cutting, chopping, and mixing. A lunch of franks and beans would be of minimal nutritional value to elderly clients, and provides virtually no tasks for participants.

Staff members closely supervise meal preparation, with one person always at the stove if hot food is being prepared. Clients are encouraged to divide tasks and cooperation is stressed. Two participants are selected to wash and dry dishes and pots while the others set the table with tablecloth, napkins, plates, utensils, and cups. Everyone eats together, with one course served at a time. A cooking group provides almost immediate gratification and has been highly successful with our population. On occasion, we have prepared sandwiches and walked to the local park for a picnic lunch.

Following lunch, the afternoon activity is based on participants' interest and energy level. We have experimented with a variety of crafts including painting, drawing, collage, clay, and holiday decorations. We also utilize structured games such as concentration and dominoes, and word games that have been simplified according to participants' abilities.

When the weather is good, the group may elect to take a walk after lunch, perhaps to look in store windows or to watch children playing in the park. At the end of the day, caregivers are given informal reports on their relatives' level of participation, and staff asks for feedback about each participant's responses at home. Often, we can assist family members in setting up an activities program for the participant at home, utilizing particular activities he enjoys while at the DAP.

SPECIAL EVENTS

Approximately once a month, participants in the day program are treated to a special event such as pet therapy or a live concert. Photographs are taken during all special events and reviewed by the group on a weekly basis. This is an additional orientation device; first, participants are reminded of activities from previous sessions, and second, identities of other group members are reinforced through photographs.

A program has been set up with Bide-A-Wee, a local humane organization, to visit the DAP with puppies and kittens (and once, a guinea pig) for our participants to enjoy. Our clients appear to enjoy cuddling, petting, and watching the antics of these animals, and often reminisce about pets they have had in the past. The participants are encouraged to feed the animals small amounts of food and bring them water to drink; this allows even the most confused client the opportunity to nurture and care for another living thing. This is particularly important at a time when the Alzheimer's victim is always receiving care from others. Following a pet therapy session, participants cut out dog and cat food coupons and we send them to the Bide-A-Wee Association, as a way of saying "thank-you" for visiting. Again, the DAP participants are doing something for the helpless animals, and at the same time benefiting from an activitiy that focuses on organization, concentration, and cooperation.

Another popular event is a live concert. An accordionist has visited the center several times. He plays songs of the 1930's and 1940's that are familiar to the DAP clients, encouraging sing-a-longs and dancing. It must be stressed that although an individual is confused he can still derive enjoyment from life.

Finally, we recently had a barbecue and invited family members of the participants to join us for lunch, followed by a violin concert. Caregivers expressed their surprise that the clients still sang and danced, and that the DAP participants had prepared salads and desserts for the barbecue. It seems that caregivers consistently underestimate the skills an Alzheimer's victim maintains.

CONCLUSION

Since the Day Activities Program at the New York Institute for Aging is less than a year old, no formal research has yet been done within our setting. Such research may be indicated in determining how our day program affects participants' functioning at home, how caregivers are assisted in coping by redirecting their family members' energy into activities, and which activities are most successful with moderately demented individuals.

It is evident to the author that occupational therapists, with their unique abilities to adapt and modify activities, should be more involved in the overall care of the Alzheimer's victim. Rehabilitative professionals need to further explore their role in maintenance therapy.

REFERENCES

1. Schneck, M. K., Reisberg, B., and Ferris, S. H.: An overview of current concepts of Alzheimer's Disease. *Am J Psychiatry* 139: 165–173, 1982.

2. Brody, E. M.: "The formal support network: Congregate treatment settings for residents with senescent brain dysfunction." In: Clinical Aspects of Alzheimer's Disease and Senile Dementia, N. Miller and G. Cohen, Eds. New York: Raven Press, 1981.

3. Mace, N. L. and Rabins, P. V.: Day care and dementia. *Generations* 9:41–45, 1984.

4. Reisberg, B., and others.: The global deterioration scale for assessment of primary degenerative dementia. *Am J Psychiatry* 139: 1136–1139, 1982.

The Selection of Activities: A Dual Responsibility

Ruth McCrum Griffin, PhD, OTR
Maureen Unger Matthews, RN, MSN

Activity selection for patients with dementia is frequently planned from a general understanding of the needs of a confused elderly population. This often leads to stereotyping of patients and inappropriate activities.

Within the context of individual and group treatment modalities, the authors discuss the value of individual patient assessment which leads to a more accurate determination of patient needs. Goals can be set for each patient and activities planned which will help the patient reach his/her goal. Consideration is given to the unique needs of patients with dementia in an extended care facility. Examples of appropriate group activities are suggested.

The selection of activities for the elderly patient suffering from one of the dementias follows basically the same process employed in the selection of activities for any patient. The added dimension of the patient's dementia may serve as either a restriction or as an expansion, depending upon the insight and creativity of the therapist.

It is the intent of the authors to discuss the process of activity selection for the elderly in general, and to focus upon those factors which may be considered unique to the elderly with dementia. The authors view activity selection from the role of the psychiatric clinical specialist and the occupational therapist.

Traditionally, the occupational therapist has been con-

Ruth McCrum Griffin, 23 Westfield Road, West Hartford, CT 06119. She is Professor of Occupational Therapy at Quinnipiac College. Maureen Unger Matthews, 23 Prospect Avenue, Norwalk, CT 06850. She is Clinical Nurse Specialist and Geropsychiatric Coordinator at the Fairfield Manor Health Care Center, Inc.

cerned with patient involvement. Therapists employed in extended care facilities have the professional responsibility of selecting areas of involvement which meet individual patient's needs; however, administrators frequently see group activities as a cost-wise more effective use of a therapist's time. The therapist is placed in the stressful situation of having to justify activity selection in terms of professional commitment concurrent with the demands of administration. This combination makes it difficult to provide the services which will satisfy both demands. Satisfaction must rest with the knowledge that benefits can be provided in both treatment situations.

The psychiatric clinical specialist in the extended care facility has been concerned with the treatment of the emotional aspects of physical disorders. For patients with dementia, this means addressing the isolation and loneliness which comes with the gradual loss of cognitive functioning combined with institutionalization. Like the occupational therapist, the nurse chooses between two treatment modalities, individual treatment and/or group treatment, the choice being dependent on the needs of the patient.

Since both therapist and nurse are planning "treatment" and not "busy work," the process for selection of activities follows the established order of patient assessment and goal setting. What is unique is the content of the activity which is geared to the functional abilities of the patient.

INDIVIDUAL TREATMENT

The primary value of individual treatment is that the patient is provided with personalized, direct attention which can respond immediately to his changing needs. The therapist also has the benefit of dealing with just one patient at a time. Despite these advantages, this treatment situation is limiting in that it prevents the therapist from seeing the patients' interaction in a group setting. Since group interaction should be included in any comprehensive type of evaluation, it is important for the therapist to be able to observe the patient in a setting with other patients.

Most therapists and nurses are better able to provide patients with a feeling of warmth and understanding on a one-to-one basis rather than in a group setting. The patient becomes the center of attention, and this focusing of attention gives the patient a sense of importance. Additionally, it may be easier to establish communication with a patient when working alone. Conversation may include more critical material than would be possible to elicit in another type of setting. The therapist may also pick up nuances impossible in a setting where others are vying for her attention. Usually rapport is established more quickly on a one-to-one basis, although this is not always the case.

Prior to selecting any type of activity when working with an individual patient, it is essential that therapist and patient have time to become acquainted and be more comfortable with one another. An initial period of "getting to know you" is important for the success of the treatment periods which are to follow. Adequate time for this process to develop should be considered an essential part of treatment. An inexperienced person may assume that this can be accomplished while working with the patient on a pre-selected activity; these authors feel that it should be a distinctly different period during which the sole purpose of the interaction is for the therapist and the patient to get to know each other.

EVALUATION

Continuing evaluation is the keynote to adapting treatment to meet the changing needs of patients. Without this, treatment can become a stagnant experience. Following the development of a relationship between patient and therapist, an initial evaluation must be completed and specific treatment goals and objectives established. If time has been taken to develop a positive relationship between patient and therapist, the evaluation is completed more easily and more accurately.

Once the initial evaluation has been completed, patient and therapist should begin to identify those problem areas to be addressed as part of the treatment process. Some elderly patients may be hesitant about being with new people and working with a therapist. A program may need to be developed which will help to overcome this difficulty. If the patient feels comfortable with the therapist and has slowly developed a feeling of trust, he may admit that this had been a life-long problem and not one which he feels is worthy of investing energy. On the other hand, it may have been a problem area which the patient has longed to change, and may gain great comfort and relief from receiving help. Superficial relationships will not usually elicit this level of information.

The time necessary to get to know the patient and develop a therapeutic relationship may cause some degree of consternation with facility administrators who do not see this as part of the treatment process. The lay individual may have difficulty equating a relaxed conversation with a process for which a charge can be made.

ACTIVITY SELECTION

The selection of individual treatment activities is, of course, dependent upon the needs of the patients. The busy therapist may assume that expressed needs exist, without realizing the importance of non-expressed needs. Since the basic tenets of occupational therapy are concerned with activities, it becomes obvious that the therapist is concerned with having the patient "do" something, which can be seen, judged or evaluated. Little value is given to encouraging the patient to do "nothing" unless it has these characteristics.

We can measure certain degrees of involvement when that involvement centers around an activity; for example, we can count how many times a patient voluntarily participated in a given activity. We cannot count or measure the degree of happiness or peace which a patient may experience when sitting quietly remembering the past. Therapists talk of the value of reminiscence therapy and of the life-review process, but many of us see these as activities which are carried out at a designated time and a set period. Remembering doesn't necessarily fall into such a neat category, but comes upon us when least expected. This may occur in the middle of a treatment session, being triggered by something which was said or done. It appears at these times that the patient has "drifted off" and the conscientious therapist immediately attempts to bring the patient back to the level of consciousness at which he was previously operating. Perhaps this is a mistake. Allowing the dementia patient time to recall past events is important; recalling them in the midst of a treatment program may be inconvenient, but that does not make them any less important. The elderly patient must remember when he is able to remember. He cannot always conjure up memories when told to do so and may thereby lose the value of the recalling process.

The elderly demented have special needs which cannot always be met within the usual structure of activities found in a nursing home setting. Activities need to be extremely flexible within given time frames. There must be totally non-structured periods where the patient is permitted to meet his own needs as he sees them.

GROUP TREATMENT

Another treatment modality which meets the needs of the cognitively impaired patient is the group. For those patients whose individual assessment reveals an interpersonal disorientation and regressive behavior, a group setting can improve their quality of life. By interpersonal disorientation we mean communication difficulties caused by a combination of losses. There is a significant language loss which makes the production of speech, as well as its understanding, difficult. There is also a loss of familiar surroundings and familiar faces. Memory loss can make even family and friends inaccessible.

Behavior changes, like interpersonal abilities, vary according to the stages of dementia, but are marked by a decreased ability to manage personal care. For these patients, a group treatment modality can meet several needs. One, it can become a *primary or reference group*. If the same five to six patients meet consistently around many types of activities, they can become "familiar faces" which they can begin to trust. When they are with people that they can trust on a basic feeling level, they do not feel judged and are more apt to perform at their highest level of functioning.

Group treatment can also address *improvement in behavior*. Patients respond to the approval and disapproval of their peers when they are part of a group they can trust. An indirect benefit from this behavior change is the effect it has on the nursing staff. When staff see a patient as having potential through the achievement of a goal within the group, they will begin to treat the patient differently outside the group. This confirms the positive behavior of the patient and allows room for continued growth, something that is not possible when patients are labeled as "problems" or benignly ignored.

Group treatment provides *repetition* of an activity which is necessary for the learning process in patients with dementia. This is true for a daily living skill group or a reality orientation group. Repetition of the same material with each patient in the group helps everyone retain the information.

SELECTING GROUP PARTICIPANTS

Selection for the group comes after individual assessments. Groups should be comprised of individuals whose functional capacities are similar. This will allow for a common goal to be attained by all members of the group through the activity planned by the therapist. This does not preclude, however, individual goals for each member of the group.

Communication styles should also be considered in the selection of patients in the group. Too many "problem" patients in a group can set a direction that was not intended in the planning.

NEED FOR ON-GOING EVALUATIONS

On-going evaluations of patients are important to determine their progress, as well as their continued appropriateness for the group. Depending on the type of dementia there can be a step-wise decline which permits a patient to function at a certain level for an indeterminate amount of time or there can be a progressive deterioration in which the patient is constantly declining in functional capacities. Care must be taken not to overstress a patient by asking him to attain a goal that is no longer within his capabilities. This can lead to agitated behavior and a catastrophic reaction.

EXAMPLES OF SUCCESSFUL ACTIVITY SELECTION

The content of the activities can be as varied as the imagination of the therapist. Groups can meet the goals of both the nurse and occupational therapist by providing content related to improving motor skills or sensory perception, while at the same time nurturing the dynamics of group interaction. One group was planned around grooming skills. With mirrors and combs, the patients fixed their own hair, had the therapist fix each person's hair and finally had patients fixing one another's hair. This group allowed for individual functional improvement and at the same time brought patients into real contact with one another.

The need for exercise is common to all, including the nursing home resident. It is possible to provide a graduated program of exercises for patients, regardless of age. This type of activity does not respond as well to individual instruction as it does to group instruction, which has the additional advantage of providing an opportunity for socialization. The residents encourage one another, provide a continuing stimulus to each other, and show a definite carry-over from an organized exercise session to their regular unit activities. The benefits of this activity can be seen in the improved posture of the residents as well as their increased ease in mobility.

SUMMARY

The key to planning activities for the elderly with dementia is the understanding that patients are at different stages in their disease and must be planned for on an individual basis. Goals must be set and evaluated at regular intervals. Both nurse and therapist participate in this on-going process of evaluation and treatment to avoid stereotyping and promote creative activity programming.

BIBLIOGRAPHY

Burnside, Irene (1978). *Working with the Elderly Group Process and Techniques.* Massachusetts Duxbury Press.
Fox, Nancy L. (1983). *How to put Joy into Geriatric Care.* St. Mary's Press; Winona, Minnesota.

Kane, Rosalie A. and Kane, Robert L. (1984). *Assessing the Elderly; A Practical Guide to Measurement*. Lexington Books; Lexington, Massachusetts.

Lewis, Carole Bernstein (1985). *Aging: The Health Care Challenge*. F. A. Davis Company; Philadelphia.

Mace, Nancy L. and Rabins, Peter V. (1981). *The 36-Hour Day*. The Johns Hopkins University Press; Baltimore.

Reisberg, Barry (1984 February). Stages of Cognitive Decline. *American Journal of Nursing*, pp 225–228.

In Search of Brain-Behavior Relationships in Dementia and the Luria-Nebraska Neuropsychological Battery

Catherine Erickson Barrett, MS, OTR, FAOTA

ABSTRACT. Attempts to localize specific brain structural changes and related associated behavior in dementia of the elderly have been plagued with theoretical and methodological controversy. There is much confusion involved in differentiating normal aging processes, healthy aging, and pathological aging. There also appears to be a loss of autonomy between physical and psychological functions in the elderly. Thus structural and functional changes noted in the elderly cannot be linked with certainty to any known or yet to be discovered normal and/or pathological processes. Researchers using the Luria-Nebraska Neuropsychological test battery are optimistic that the instrument may be useful in delineating normal from abnormal brain structures and related neuropsychological functions in the elderly. The battery also furnishes clinicians with opportunities to establish baseline behaviors, make decisions based on quantifiable data, and evaluate the efficacy of their treatments. Therapists of various disciplines, social scientists and other are encouraged to integrate their discipline specific knowledge bases with neuropsychological findings. This might lead to inter and intra disciplinary solutions to problems shared in common and/or unique to each discipline. The LNNB is discussed in detail with common findings in dementia indicated and implications for therapy, education and research presented.

Catherine Erickson Barrett, Assistant Professor, Department of Occupational Therapy, IN Central University, 1400 East Hanna Avenue, Indianapolis, IN 46227 (317) 788-3429, and Consultant, Indianapolis Jewish Home for the Aged, Inc. (Hooverwood), Indianapolis, IN 46260.

I gratefully acknowledge the support and assistance of Dr. Dotty Weeks and Sandy Clark of Indiana Central University as well as the staff, residents, and family members of Hooverwood who allowed me to expand my horizons.

Ever since Herophilius of Chalcedon (300 B.C.) attempted to localize cognitive functions in the ventricular cavities of the brain, localizationists have searched for linkages between isolated brain structures and specific functional abilities. It is believed that knowledge of specific brain structural damage could explain a specific functional loss and vice versa. A divergent group, the equipotentialists, view the brain as an undifferentiated whole and behavior as completely dependent upon the brain's integrity and its holistic interdependent processes. These molar viewers of the brain argue that impairment of higher cognitive functions cannot be attributed to any specific molecular brain damage area but rather to the total amount of brain tissue involved regardless of location. Some, such as Kurt Goldstein, believe that brain damage not only affects abstract thinking and personality, but also adaptive response toward self-realization and meaningful existence (Golden, 1981; Hartlage & DeFilippis, 1983).

The following summarizes some of the current knowledge of brain-behavior relationships in dementia with emphasis on the Luria-Nebraska Neuropsychological Battery (LNNB). This knowledge and the use of such instruments as LNNB can assist therapists of various disciplines, social scientists and others working with victims of dementia to find intra and inter disciplinary solutions to problems shared in common and/or unique to each discipline.

DEMENTIA AND BRAIN PATHOLOGY

Present day localizationists and equipotentialists are especially challenged by the increasing prevalence of dementia among our ever growing elderly population. Dementia is caused by a number of known and unknown factors which affect the brain and its functions. This diagnosis is "warranted only if intellectual deterioration is of sufficient severity to interfere with social or occupational functioning." "Dementia is *not* synonymous with aging" (American Psychiatric Association, 1980, p. 110), although the risk for dementing disorders increases after 65. Depending upon source and definition used, those 85 or older have a 20–50% chance of developing dementia (Cohen, 1982; Kay & Bergmann, 1980).

There are similarities in both the structural and functional changes in the brains of older non-demented individuals and those suffering from degenerative dementia (Price, 1980; Sloane, 1980; Swendseid, 1982; Habot & Libow, 1980). Symptoms of dementia may occur in the absence of known brain pathology and, likewise, degenerative brain changes may be present without any accompanying behavioral disorder(s) (Drachman, 1980; MacInnes, 1981; Ochsner, 1976). Some functional disorders, especially depression, common in the elderly, produce symptoms often seen in dementia. Some may mask, mimic, or, as with paranoid disorders, even complicate and accelerate changes in the early stages of dementing illnesses (Miller, 1980; Post, 1980).

Of the elderly suffering from severe intellectual impairments, 10–20% are estimated to have any of more than 100 illnesses, curable or partially treatable by means of medical, nutritional, and/or environmental intervention. Most of the remaining 80% are considered irreversible or progressively degenerative and incurable at this time. These are attributed primarily to senile dementia of the Alzheimer's type and, to a lesser degree to multi-infarct diseases or to a combination of Alzheimer's and multi-infarct dementia (NIA Task Force, 1980; NIA, 1983; NIH, 1981).

SIMPLE TASKS AND FUNCTIONAL SYSTEMS

Russian neuropsychologist, A. R. Luria conceived of the brain as a whole made up of functional systems, thus offering an alternative approach to the difficult but crucial task of differentiating brain structural and functional changes resulting from normal aging and those resulting from dementing illnesses. Luria, who developed his theories in the 1960's, incorporated elements of the localizationists and the equipotentialists. He retained the concept of local cortical areas mediating specific skills but at a very elementary level. Thus any simple task could involve a multitude of cortical sites requiring joint work of different levels and brain areas (Golden, 1981).

Luria separated the brain into three basic blocks, each specialized but working together as a team. The first block, "energy and tone," includes the upper brain stem, reticular formation, part of the limbic cortex and hippocampus. This block is responsible for the stable tone of the cortex and for the state of vigilance or attention. The second block, "input, re-coding, and storage of information," includes the posterior parts of the hemispheres with the occipital, parietal, and temporal regions and their underlying structures. The systems of this block receive integrate and analyze proprioceptive and sensory stimuli. They are hierarchical and highly modality-specific. The third block, "frontal lobes," is not modality-specific and is important in planning, executing, and controlling one's behavior (Golden, 1981; Luria, 1969). All behavior requires the interaction of these basic blocks. Similar to the equipotential theory, the brain operates as a whole, and in accordance with localizationist theory, each area within the brain plays a specific role in each behavior.

Since variations are possible in any given task, alternative functional systems could by used to compensate for any structural loss. Higher mental functions are not viewed as unitary abilities but made up of varying numbers of simpler and more basic skills, each of which involves a different functional system (Golden, 1981; Luria, 1969; McInnes, 1983a). Such a theory might be used to explain why some individuals with severe brain dysfunction are still able to function with minimal behavioral impairment. Pathological processes could have developed slowly, with continual compensation or establishment of new functional systems with each structural change. Thus identification of remaining elementary skills could assist clinicians in choosing appropriate communication systems and/or retraining to establish alternative functional systems.

Despite the volumes written about intelligence, very few authorities agree on its definition. When the word intelligence is used in reference to the elderly, contradictory conclusions are made. Numerous studies report that test scores on psychometric devices measuring mental ability decline with age. An equal number of studies could be cited which conclude that intelligence remains stable with age, and performance on testing depends upon the effects of educational-cultural experiences and not age per se. Some studies indicate an actual increase in certain intellectual functions, expecially in older women's verbal scores and older men's arithmetic scores (Bischof, 1976). Other studies indicate that decline is not noticeable until the 80's or 90's (Botwinick, 1973; Gillen et al., 1982) while some see only a "terminal drop" or abrupt decline just shortly before death (Bischof, 1976; Botwinick, 1973).

It would appear that intelligence is not a unitary function but one composed of many component sub-skills and influenced by many factors. Test results would therefore depend on the psychometric device used, scoring and interpretation basis, the educational-cultural experiences of both the testers and testees, and other known and unknown factors.

Raymond B. Cattel introduced the concepts of fluid and crystallized intelligence to explain some of the contradictory findings (Cattel, 1965). Fluid intelligence is primarily innate and involves all types of problem-solving, flexibility, and creative insight. It reaches maturity between the ages of 14–16. It is used in formulating and understanding series, classifications, analogies, and complex relations. It appears unconnected with cultural skills and is affected by brain injury in any area. Crystallized intelligence consists of reasoning, mechanical information and skills, social judgment, vocabulary and numerical ability. Isolated components are affected depending upon specific area brain damage with the rest remaining intact. Repeatedly the younger adults score higher than older adults on items measuring fluid memory and the older better than the younger on items measuring crystallized intelligence (Bischof, 1976; Cattel, 1965; McInnes, 1981; Swendreid, 1982).

Such findings may substantiate the assumption that intellectual decline is *not* the consequence of normal aging process but of some other factor(s). Significant cognitive deterioration seen in dementia most likely represents changes in brain functioning that are qualitatively different from those caused by the normal process of aging (Gillen et al., 1982). There also appears to be the possibility that different brain functions as well as different brain regions are affected by aging at different rates. Whether such differential aging can be attributed to normal aging processes, disease processes, or other factors is still not clear (Botwinick, 1973; Cohen, 1982; Goldstein, 1983; Swendseid, 1982; Zarit, 1978).

MEMORY AND CELL ASSEMBLIES

Most studies seem to report short-term memory decline with age. This decline may be linear or abrupt and more often involves recall rather than recognition (Bischof, 1976: Botwinick, 1973). Loss of memory appears to be the most common complaint in the early stages of dementing illnesses. Memory is closely linked to learning in that learning also involves trace formation (input, stimulus response, registering), storage (memory trace, neural connections), and utilization of retrieval (recognition or recall). There is indication that memory, like intelligence, involves many component parts. For instance, one can speak of a musician's auditory memory, a policeman's visual memory, and an athlete's kinesthetic memory. Since visual retention has been said to decline with age (Bischof, 1976), measurement of memory or learning utilizing only visual stimuli may be invalid.

There are differences of opinion as to whether one or more neuronal mechanisms are involved in memory trace formation. The unitary-mechanism theorists view short-term and long-term memory as one continuum. The two-mechanism theory can be represented by Donald O. Hebb's hypothetical "cell assemblies," supposedly spread over widely dispersed cortical areas (Hebb, 1945, 1966). The activity in one cell facilitates activity of the others within that cell assembly. There is, therefore, a reverberating activity from one cell to the next as in a closed circuit after the original stimulation has ceased. This activity decays rapidly and is extremely vulnerable to interference such as the introduction of new stimuli. This first phase, "dynamic phase" is said to be the basis for short-term memory. A second phase, "static phase," occurs when recurring reverberating activity results in structural changes at the synapses or formation of synaptic knobs (since this is only a theory, no consistent time factor has been identified). This enduring biochemical state results in memory consolidation and is the basis for long-term memory. The greater the number and size of synaptic knobs, the greater the facilitatory capacity of a cell to stimulate another cell in its cell assembly as well as a cell in another cell assembly. Each cell assembly is said to represent a single image or percept. Several cell assemblies become associated so that more complex concepts can be recalled (Hebb, 1945, 1966).

The above descriptions of coordinated efforts are similar to groups of functional systems involved in one task. In the case of dementia, it would appear that repetitive stimulation of already existing cell assemblies or repetition of previously learned percepts and concepts would have the greatest chance of facilitating memories and learned behaviors. The utilization and retrieval of stored memories depend upon a variety of factors. Some believe that recognition memory does not require retrieval as does recall memory. It is difficult to distinguish between dysfunction in ability to retrieve memories and deficiencies in the storage system itself.

Localizationists have attempted to link the left hippocampal gyrus with verbal memory and right hippocampal gyrus with spatial memory. Bilateral involvement may lead to the complete loss of recent memory (Golden, 1981). In Alzheimer's disease, neurofibrillary tangles are found in the cerebral cortex and are especially concentrated in the pyramidal cells of the hippocampus. These neurofibrils are present in non-demented elderly but in much lesser density and distribution (Reisberg, 1981). Such findings support the current practice of using familiar consistent routines in a familiar environment with dementia victims who have lost ability to store new data and recall recent events. The concept of decaying reverberating circuits may be involved in explaining the severely demented individual's inconsistent ability to attempt a correct response within a second or two of stimulus. Lack of ability to make connection with other cell assemblies would seem to prevent retrieval of concepts and organization to execute a planned response. Perhaps simple recognition is involved.

NORMAL, HEALTHY AND PATHOLOGICAL AGING

Accurate and early identification and differentiation of normal aging processes, treatable disorders, and degenerative dementia are crucial in order to avoid self-fulfilling prophecies of decline and therapeutic nihilism (Eisdorfer et al., 1981; Miller, 1980; Price et al., 1980; Spinaris-Attrel, 1979; Zarit et al., 1981). Unfortunately, there are many probable known and unknown complexities of interrelated factors which make this difficult, inevitably resulting in misdiagnosis and inappropriate management. Many of these factors involve methodological research problems encountered in attempting to differentiate among "normal," "abnormal," and "healthy" aging.

In order to identify patterns of normal aging, a large heterogeneous group of aged people who have survived a wide range of physical and psychological experiences is required. This group of "normal" subjects must then be subdivided into an "abnormal" aging group and a "healthy" aging group. This in itself is difficult since we have no clear definition of healthy aging, although many biological, psychological, and sociological theories and philosophical treaties have been expounded. Most research studies involving healthy aged subjects appear to have chosen such measurable criteria as: lack of known medical and psychological conditions; freedom from stress and toxins; "healthy" nutritional habits (Goldstein, 1983); quality of personal and social support systems (Eisdorfer, 1981); subjective states of happiness, morale, and well being (Kane & Kane, 1983) and ability to function successfully in one's own environment (Kane & Kane, 1983; Patterson, 1982). Even so, all studies comparing younger healthy adults with institutionalized "healthy" but inactive, older adults, show so-called age differences (Botwinick, 1973). To simply eliminate known disease as a factor in identifying healthy adults would decrease the population to 95% of all younger adults but only 50% of the still surviving elderly adults (Schaie, 1977). Furthermore, there is the problem posed by the higher proportion of women than of men among the elderly and the tendency for women to retain their health longer than men. An experimental design incorporating equal numbers of men and women does not accurately reflect actual proportions respective to age and health. Such designs further limit cohort samples due to the difficulty in locating healthy older male volunteers (Krauss, 1980).

Research designs can also have critical impact upon the attempt to establish age-appropriate norms (Botwinick, 1977; Habot & Libow, 1980.) This involves identifying *age effects* or phenomena directly associated with chronological age; *age changes* or alterations of structure or function over time in the same individual; *age correlation* or statistically significant relations between functions or structures and chronological age in groups; and *age differences* or the variations in function or structure among various age groups (Goldstein, 1983).

While age differences among various age groups are addressed in cross-sectional research designs, age change within individuals across time are not. Age declines may be magnified because of variations in the rates of cumulative trauma from one generation to the next and because of variations in cultural and educational experiences (Botwinick, 1977; Goldstein, 1983; McInnes, 1983a; Schaie, 1977). Tests validated in one time period may not be valid in a later time period. If subpopulations are matched for education, socio-economic status, presence or absence of pathology, or institutionalization, their representativeness of the total population from which they have been drawn is severely limited (Schaie, 1977). Fewer older cohort samples are available due to: selective mortality; family members refusing to allow research; illness and confusion making testing difficult and even impossible; and limited number of qualified testers able to interact with the very old (Streib, 1983).

In longitudinal designs, patterns across the same individual over time may be examined but such research is time consuming, costly, and involves the problems of cohort attrition, socio-cultural changes from generation to generation, repeated testing, and instrumentation change. Validity of psychometric devices with one age cohort does not necessarily assure validity in measuring the same constructs in another age cohort (Schaie, 1977). Age-related patterns are minimized because of differential drop-out rates. Healthier and more intelligent persons tend to live longer. Each re-test increases bias as the age of the subsample increases (Botwinick, 1977; Goldstein, 1983). Number of volunteer subjects is limited due to income, mobility, and health factors. Even if transportation and financial inducement were involved, bias would still prevent generalization. Examiners must monitor developing concurrent and potentially confounding diseases and medical treatment (Streib, 1983). Goldstein (1983) suggests the use of a combination of both cross-sectional and longitudinal studies to differentiate dementing processes from those of normal aging.

Another methodological problem involves the testing instruments available. Often they are inappropriately chosen and administered with little regard given to their validity, reliability, item content, and administration and scoring procedures (Kane & Kane, 1983; Botwinick, 1973). Many testing instruments which can successfully identify cognitive deterioration in the moderate to severe cannot reliably detect mild or early deterioration. Because of the absence of norms for the elderly, instruments which are relatively accurate in detection of brain dysfunction in younger adults tend to have excessively high false positive rates with elderly individuals. The same test item may not be measuring the same construct in both young and elderly adults. The elderly may miss items because of decreased visual and/or auditory acuity; misunderstanding of the question due to language or educational/cultural differences; not enough response time; lack of familiarity due to life-style differences affecting relevance; motivation; rhythmic biological cycles; faulty testee-tester interaction; testing anxiety; medication side-effect; and numerous other factors confounding test performance (Habot & Libow, 1980; Schaie, 1977; Streib, 1973).

Traditional group comparison studies limit the number of variables observed and often obscure complex interrelationships involved (Spiers, 1982). Even though dementia in the elderly is a multi-faceted problem requiring multi–disciplinary solutions, we find medical model literature focusing upon the assessment, etiology, disease progression, risk factors, prevalence, and pharmaceutical management. Social model literature emphasizes environmental manipulation, support groups, life satisfaction, and interpersonal relationships. Memory, intellectual function, response time, behavior modification, and perception are emphasized in learning model literature (Patterson, 1982). Because of this fragmented search, any functional and/or structural change identified often cannot be attributed with certainty to normal aging or any specific neurological bio-chemical, viral, immunological, toxic, hereditary, psychological, social, or environmental factors (Habot & Libow, 1980).

It is rare to find a therapist who can integrate all the material from various disciplines and even more rare to find one who can translate it into practical information. There appears to be very little, relatively speaking, about the comprehensive remediation or amelioration of dementia and its associated trauma to family members and society in general (Eisdorfer, 1981; Eisdorfer et al., 1981). Clinicians must pool their areas of expertise with those of other disciplines and integrate one another's findings until the gaps of knowledge disappear. This means learning to read the jargon of various disciplines, literatures and learning to translate one's own jargon so that others could likewise benefit. It involves taking time out of busy clinical schedules to keep accurate detailed records and willingness to carry out simple research studies. Whereas one alone may not be able to find funding or time to support extensive data collection, several from different disciplines working on narrower components might find the means to do so (Feinberg, 1980). By working together in a coordinated manner with a common goal, much like the concept of functional systems, everyone involved in the present and in the future has a chance to benefit.

NEUROPSYCHOLOGY AND THE THERAPIES

Neuropsychology is a relatively new science. As a pure science, its main goal is to use sophisticated scientific methods to measure changes in specific brain structures and the associated effects on specific behaviors, especially information-processing capacities. As a clinical science, it attempts to establish levels of information-processing skills required for ability to function in society (Feinberg et al., 1980). Neuropsychologists are making important contributions in: screening for suspected brain damage; analyzing extent of deficits for legal, rehabilitation, or treatment considerations; assessing results of treatment; mapping various types of brain damage across populations; testing theoretical propositions about human brain function; and confirming, expanding, and modifying assumptions about brain-behavior relationships (Gillen et al., 1982; Golden et al., 1982). Therapists working with the elderly could expand their own skills and knowledge by integrating neuropsychological findings into their practice and research. For instance, occupational therapists, using their discipline's concepts of developmental tasks and activity analysis could further develop their science of human occupation and further explore their theories about body-mind-spiritual-social interdependency. Physical therapists, music therapists, speech therapists, dance therapists, recreational therapists, art therapists, and others could likewise find much to expand and clarify their own knowledge bases. Some, like the localizationists, may choose to deal with limited specific areas; others may adopt a more holistic viewpoint like the equipotentialists, and the rest a combination of the two.

THE LURIA-NEBRASKA
NEUROPSYCHOLOGICAL BATTERY

Therapists may discover much relevant material in the Luria-Nebraska Neuropsychological Battery, based on Luria's theories of brain-behavior relationships. Its developers have been thorough in avoiding many of the methodological pitfalls mentioned in their attempts to validate the battery across diagnostic categories and more recently in establishing age-related norms for the elderly. Because of this, the battery is being used to differentiate among so-called healthy aged, medically ill aged, emotionally ill aged, and those that suffer from various stages of dementia. It is a neuropsychological tool, but could possibly be used by specially trained and qualified professionals in other fields, thus expanding its versatility. Some of the items are similar in administration to items on the Southern California Sensory Integration Tests, Clinical Observation Scales, and other sensory, cognitive, and perceptual-motor tests commonly used in occupational therapy practice.

Luria's clinical approach was entirely qualitative. Much like many physical and occupational therapists, he used a flexible approach to assessment. This means that the results and interpretation of performance are dependent upon the skill and sophistication of the examiner. Tests and skills to be assessed are chosen, often spontaneously, by the clinician on the basis of subjective impression, available objective information, and on intuition. Approaches differ from testing situation to testing situation and deficits not considered are often overlooked. It is impossible to differentiate between the merits of the procedures used and those of the clinician's skills. Meaningful accumulation of a data base regarding the assessment procedures or testing results are not possible (Gillen, 1982; Golden et al., 1982a; Moses, 1983a). On the other hand, standardized or quantitative testing involves "actuarial" (rather than descriptive) methodologies based on normal distribution statistics and group comparisons (Spiers, 1981). Luria was opposed to standardized testing on the basis that it does not allow freedom to explore unique areas of concern.

Nevertheless, Anne-Lise Christensen in 1975 published a series of test items which closely approximated some of Luria's techniques (Moses, 1983a). In the late 1970's Golden and his associates (1983) began to work on modifying Christensen's flexible items into a standardized battery that allows some flexibility. Critics of the battery lament the loss of Luria's original flexible approach and point out difficulties involved in its administration and scoring with unique cases due to the standardization protocol and/or artificial constructional restrictions (Crosson, 1982; Delis & Kaplan, 1982; Spiers, 1981, 1982).

Attempts have been made to retain the original intent of items, and a mixture of both simple and complex items representing Luria's functional system are incorporated. Emphasis is placed on identification of the skills rather than identification of impairment of specific functional systems. Qualitative observations are also retained by allowing some flexibility in protocol and the use of "testing-the-limits" procedures, which are useful in interpretations of standard scores (Bryant et al., 1984; Golden et al., 1982b, 1983c; Moses, 1983a). Verbal instructions may be modified to fit patient's understanding except for items involving receptive speech measurements. Non-verbal responses are permitted except for expressive speech items. Other modifications are permitted as long as the intent of each item is not violated (Golden et al., 1982a, 1983). The mode of presentation and response is systematically varied within the test to differentiate among a wide range of impairments (Golden et al., 1982b).

The battery now consists of 269 items and takes approximately 2 1/2 hours to administer. This can be done in a series of sessions of varying lengths depending on fatigue tolerance. Scoring is relatively simple since each item attempts to measure a different discrete task involving a limited number of functions and minimal number of areas within each unit of the brain. Errors can be traced to relatively few possibilities. With the objective guidelines provided, one can easily distinguish among scores of "O" no deficit, "1" borderline deficit or "2" significant deficit (Golden, 1981; Golden et al., 1982, 1983).

The items are divided into 14 sub-scales representing behavioral and regional divisions. Interpretation can be made by analyzing a summation score, individual scale scores, and/ or by individual item analysis. Qualitative observations are also considered, as well as eight cortical localization scales and 30 factor scales derived from analysis of various items throughout the battery (Golden, 1981; Golden et al., 1982a, 1983; Moses, 1983b). Such analysis is quickly done by means of interpretation of computer summaries and incorporation of qualitative observations. Non-neuropsychologists are more likely to interpret results at a behavioral level whereas neuropsychologists will attempt to determine causes for performance and to localize brain structures involved (Moses et al., 1983a).

To correct for effects of age and education on test performance, raw scores are translated into T-scores and a formula is used to calculate brain impairment T-score cutoff. Brain damage is indicated when at least three scales are elevated above this individualized critical cutoff level. Education may not be as important as occupational history in determining the critical cutoff level. Many elderly have achieved high success despite lower education. The critical cutoff level may underestimate expected performance in the elderly. If scores are more than 20 points below the critical cutoff level, then the level is probably too high. One must then re-examine the occupational history. Patients who score low normal with a history of occupational success may be suffering from a subtle decline. This decline may not be obvious on first testing due to pre-morbid above-average abilities. A second testing within a year will usually pick up a decline of such a subtle nature (Golden et al., 1983; Malloy, 1981).

Table 1 presents a summary of the clinical scales and some selected findings regarding performance by elderly individuals with dementia. In the case of very impaired demented individuals, it is quite difficult to make specific conclusions about

Table 1

Clinical Scales of the Luria-Nebraska Neuropsychological Battery

Scale	Stimuli	Functions Involved	Dementia Findings
Motor	Verbal command Visual cues Demonstration Practice	Hand, mouth, tongue Visuo-spatial tasks Kinesthetic feedback Speed & coordination Recept. Speech Vision	Loss of complex & sequential movement Better at copying than drawing from verbal cue Area least affected in early stages
Rhythm	Audio	Vocalization of pitch Discrimination of tones Duplicate rhythm Receptive speech Expressive speech Motor skills Hearing	Able to hum & sing Maintain simple rhythmic pattern Environmental sounds a problem
Tactile	Verbal commands Soft, hard, blunt sharp stimuli 2-point stimuli Ipsilateral arm positioning Common objects Moving touch	Soft, hard, blunt, sharp discrimination Graphesthesia Limb position in space Kinesthetic feedback 2-point discrimination Stereognosis Receptive speech	Less sensory loss than motor Receptive speech is a problem Many resist being blindfolded-use alternative method Adapt for motor deficits
Visual	Simple objects Pictures Overlapped designs Clock faces Compass faces Block designs Rotated designs	Visual-spatial perception Recognition Word finding Figure-ground Spatial rotation Receptive speech Expressive speech	Aphasia is a problem Poor vision a problem in determining visual-spatial skills
Receptive	Phonemes Syllables Sequenced sounds Verbal commands	Phonemic discrimination Phonemic production Comprehension of words, phrases, sentences Constructional motor planning Writing Recall Expressive speech Vision & Hearing Body-part identification	Greater loss than expressive speech Area of second greatest loss Ill fitting dentures a problem Hearing loss a problem
Expressive	Verbal & written phonemes, words, sentences Picture Audio story Missing work printed sentence Printed jumbled words	Articulation of phonemes words & sentences of increasing complexity Automatic sequences Spontaneous speech Recognizing words Retrieval of missing word Sequencing Syntactic skills Verbal fluency Immediate memory Receptive speech	Correct responses first section Ill fitting dentures a problem Hearing loss a problem

TABLE 1 (continued)

Scale	Stimuli	Functions Involved	Dementia Findings
Writing	Verbal command Dictation Visual (letters, words)	Copy letters, syllables Write from dictation Write from thoughts Receptive speech Vision	Most intact area

Reading	Visual (letters, words, sentences)
	Verbal commands
		Reading of phonemes
		    words, phrases &
		    paragraphs
		Analyze words
		Synthesize words
			Fair number of losses
			Difficult to separate
			    deficits in oral
			    expression from reading
			    comprehension

Arithmetic	Dictation
	Arabic numerals
	Roman numerals
	Simple problems
	Verbal commands
		Identification of Arabic
		    & Roman numerals
		Comparison of numbers
		Perform simple arithmetic
		    operations
		Perform serial subtraction
		Vision
		Receptive speech
			Area of greatest loss
			Associated with frontal
			    deficits
			Test anxiety a problem
			    for the more normal

Memory	Verbal cues &
	    commands
	Pictures
	Rhythmic patterns
	Hand positions
		Immediate memory of
		    verbal, visual,
		    acoustic, &
		    kinesthetic stimuli
		Retractive & proactive
		    interference effects
		Color discrimination
		Vision & Speech
		Picture paired associated
		    tasks
			First area elevated in
			    early stages
			Associated with temporal
			    deficits

Intellect.
Functions
	Pictures
	Verbal commands
	Dictated story
	Proverbs
		Interpretation of orally
		    presented stories
		Interpretation of
		    pictures
		Picture arrangement
		Proverb interpretation
		Classification
		Formation of analogies
		Complex math problems
		Sequencing ability
		Color discrimination
		Humor
		Vision & speech
			Area of third
			    greatest loss
			Associated with
			    temporal deficits

Pathogno-
metic Scale
	NA
	Calculated from
	    scores on 34
	    items
		Seriousness & acuteness
		    of brain dysfunction
			Elevated scores

Right
Hemisphere
	NA
	Calculated from 21
	    motor & tactile
	    items
		Measure of lateralization
		
		Left hand sensory & motor
		    functions
			Diffuse brain damage
			    average score 41
			    (normal 22, S.D. 9)
			Slightly greater
			    involvement than left
			    hemisphere

Left
Hemisphere
	NA
	Calculated from 21
	    motor & tactile
	    items
		Measure of Laterali-
		    zation
		Right hand sensory
		    & motor functions
			Diffuse brain damage
			    average score 36
			    (normal 16, S.D., 9)
			Associated with left
			    sensorimotor deficits

visual, tactile, and other areas due to their inability to follow any instructions or initiate behavior in response to outside requests or stimuli. It is also difficult to reach conclusions about nonverbal skills in the case of severe global aphasics (Moses et al., 1983).

The eight localization scales include analysis of those items which are associated with either the right or left frontal lobes, temporal lobes, parietal-occipital areas and sensorimotor areas. Average LNNB performance of elderly individuals with dementia indicates that the greatest area of dysfunction is shown by the right parietal-occipital scale (RPO) and second most affected are by the left parietal-occipital scale (LPO). The RPO is involved in spatial functions and constructional activities. The LPO is involved with logical grammatical transformation and word finding and is highly related to educational achievement (Gillen et al., 1982). Since there is, in general, a diffuse brain involvement with this population, these scales are used only to generate hypotheses about the deficits. If two of the eight localization scales are above the critical level, there is evidence for brain damage (Moses et al., 1983a, 1983b).

The least reliable aspect of the LNNB (.75 as opposed to .88 for the clinical and localization scales) are the 30 factor scales, due to the low numbers of items per scale. Nevertheless, the profiles and analysis of elementary skills which they provide are useful supplementary data when interpreted cautiously. These scores are useful in syndrome analysis, providing profile patterns associated with various types of brain damage (Moses et al., 1983a). The most affected factor scales among 35 demented subjects were the motor writing skills, number reading, and verbal-spatial relationship (Gillen et al., 1982). (See Table 2.)

Reynolds (1982) proposed the use of ipsative test score interpretation in addition to the normative approach with the LNNB. This approach allows one to assess intra-individual differences in performance. By comparing performance scores with one's own unique mean level rather than normed standards, one might be able to calculate minute changes not otherwise obvious. Standard scores on the 11 subscales are averaged permitting the comparison of each subtest score with this number. This difference will either be above average

Table 2

Factor Scales of the Luria-Nebraska Neuropsychology Battery

M1	Kinesthesis-Based Movements	Rh1	Rhythm & Pitch Perception
M2	Drawing Speed	E1	Simple Phonetic Reading
M3	Fine Motor Speed	E2	Word Repetition
M4	Spatial-Based Movement	E3	Reading Poly-Syllables
M5	Oral Motor Skills	Rg1	Reading Complex Material
T1	Simple Tactile Sensation	Rg2	Reading Simple Material
T2	Stereognosis	W1	Spelling
V1	Visual Acuity & Naming	W2	Motor Writing Skill
V2	Visual-Spatial Organization	A1	Arithmetic Calculations
Rc1	Phonemic Discrimination	A2	Number Reading
Rc2	Relational Concepts	Me1	Verbal Memory
Rc3	Concept Recognition	Me2	Visual & Complex Memory
Rc4	Verbal-Spatial Relations	I1	General Verbal Intelligence
Rc5	Word Comprehension	I2	Complex Verbal Arithmetic
Rc6	Logical Grammatical Relations	I3	Simple Verbal Arithmetic

or below average regardless of normed standards. It is possible to calculate the standard error of the difference between a subscale score and the mean of all subscales.

Healthy older adults have scored within one standard deviation of the original Battery control group (McInnes et al., 1982, 1984; Spitzform, 1982). In one sample only 8% scored at a level indicative of brain damage. There were significant age-effects on 11 of the 14 clinical scales but differences noted were qualitatively different from the performance of a group of demented elderly. Men tended to do better on the visual scale and women better on the expressive speech and pathognomonic scale. When comparing performance between the younger healthy aged subjects and the older healthy aged subjects, the older group performed *better* on the writing and expressive speech scales (McInnes et al., 1981, 1982). When compared to younger healthy adults, the older healthy adults performed at a slightly lower level (McInnes et al., 1984).

Highly significant differences were found between a group

of healthy aged subjects and a group of brain-damaged elderly which included those with dementing illnesses. The brain damaged group scored worse on all scales except writing. Profiles correctly classified 92% of the healthy elderly ($\bar{x}$ = 71 years) and 86% of the brain damaged elderly ($\bar{x}$ = 68 years). There is concern that some who score in the normal range may actually have subtle decline, especially if pre-morbidly superior. Repeated testing may be necessary (McInnes et al., 1984).

In a mixed group made up of both healthy and demented elderly, decrements in performance on the battery paralleled decrements in the gray matter blood flow. There was a much lesser relationship between white matter blood flow and performance. The regional blood flow (rCBF) was lower in the mixed group of elderly when compared to that of a healthy group. The rCBF accounted for approximately 13–30% of the variance on performance of the LNNB (McInnes & Quaile, 1982). Differences in some radiological measures paralleled differences on the battery. There was a general relationship between ventricular measurements and LNNB scores whereas relationships between measurements of brain atrophy and poorer performance on the LNNB were limited. There appeared to be some relationship between tactile and receptive language skills and density changes in the anterior measurements. There was significant relationship between overall functional levels and CT scan measures of cortical atrophy but none between specific cognitive tasks and measures of cortical atrophy (McInnes, Franzen, & Mahoney, 1983).

When compared to the Halstead-Reitan, the LNNB was able to better identify brain-damaged patients from those with psychiatric disorders (Kane et al., 1981). Mildly to moderately depressed individuals score within normal limits on the LNNB. The consistent pattern associated with demented individuals is not seen in depressed elderly.

Individuals in the early stages of Alzheimer's Disease demonstrate difficulties across several scales. Memory, receptive speech, arithmetic, intellectual and rhythm scales. With a repeat testing in six to twelve months, these findings can be differentiated from deficits due to depression even in premorbidly very bright individuals.

IMPLICATIONS FOR THERAPISTS

In Assessment Tool Development

Therapists attempting to develop their own instruments could gain forewarning of the pitfalls of both standardized and subjective assessment by reading about the LNNB. The literature, both in praise of and in criticism of LNNB, may help therapists in the planning and development stages of validating a new instrument. Such literature may provide a model for overcoming obstacles, errors, and criticisms. The literature may even help increase their appreciation of intra-professional criticism and controversy as a sign of professional growth. On a more practical level, the literature may provide some of the rationale for theoretical foundations required in their instrument development.

In Treatment Planning and Implementation

We are told that only the physician can diagnose. Yet therapists working in geriatric settings are expected to "treat" patients with diagnoses of senility, organic brain syndrome, hip fracture, CVA, dehydration, malnutrition, etc., with little other information. Often the diagnoses and occasionally even the medical history omit mentioning psychological components due to reimbursement problems. Therapists must convince Medicaid officials and other third party payers that their services are resulting in some form of measurable improvement. Maintaining function is no longer viewed as improvement even in the case of degenerating illnesses.

A tool such as the LNNB could help therapists and the rest of the medical team establish concrete baselines from which to establish priorities. Information regarding a patient's neuropsychological functioning in addition to medical and social histories would be helpful in choosing the most effective management strategy and assignment to units and programs. Perhaps the most valuable aspect of this information to health care professionals and other caretakers would be the identification of remaining strengths. Knowing how to communicate (which syntax to use, length of phrases, grammar, etc.) with a severely demented individual may offer an alternative to restraints. Knowing which stimuli have the greatest possibility of facilitating positive responses for a particular individual would help maintain independence in some functional areas and in choosing optimal environmental factors such as colors, sounds, smells, types of activities, amount of social interaction, types of auditory or visual cues and timing of routine activities.

In Treatment Comparison Studies

Many of the assessment tools used by therapists lack sensitivity to measure the very aspects they intuitively believe indicate "improvement." In several therapeutic services comparison studies using the questionable assessment tools, the authors concluded they found no significant differences. Yet in the discussion sections, they described staff's observation of patients' increase in length and amount of verbalization, wider range of affect, increased fluidity and coordination in movements, increase in attention span and various other behaviors not measured by the instruments used. An instrument such as the LNNB could take the more global indicators of improvement and provide quantifiable measurement of some of their component parts.

The LNNB could be administered to a sample of patients; the treatment(s) provided to a random sub-sample and routine activities to the rest (a control group) for an appropriate length of time based on the treatment requirements and/or reimbursement regulations regarding number of allowable sessions; and the Form II version of the LNNB re-administered following this time and possibly six months later for a post post-testing. Simple statistics could be used to analyze differences in the mean scores of the groups before and after the treatment(s). The post post-test scores could further indicate the lasting effects of the treatment and give opportunity to measure differences in rate of degeneration. The battery's sensitivity could allow quantifiable and qualitative conclusions to be made about such behaviors as response time, speech patterns, motor skills, attention span, auditory and visual retention, etc.

In Program Effectiveness Studies

As our elderly population continues to grow in numbers and in age, the incidence of progressive dementing illnesses is expected to also increase. The public is demanding effective treatment; government officials are desperately seeking effective treatment and cost-efficient comprehensive services. Therapists have the skills, knowledge, and potential to make a tremendous contribution in the management of dementing illnesses. Some of the therapies already possess the holistic philosophies or wide-based perspective so necessary in this area. The LNNB could be used to show differences in rate of degeneration between those who receive various therapies and those who do not. The process could concomitantly provide useful data to help decision-makers plan, develop, and implement therapeutic and/or rehabilitative programs.

In Behavior Analysis

Each of the therapies appears to be concerned with a limited domain of behaviors related to their discipline's modalities and training background. Experienced practitioners often analyze these behaviors unconsciously in order to spontaneously alter intervention strategies as needed. Despite guidelines given, students often have difficulty differentiating between relevant and irrelevant factors when attempting to make clinical decisions based on observation of behaviors. Their role models often have difficulty explaining in words what they do more or less intuitively. Studying the concept of Luria's functional systems and the LNNB could give students a greater understanding and appreciation of the complexity of the simplest act. It might even help students explain why a certain patient has difficulty performing one task and not another. Students would become more aware of the importance of the nature of their verbal, visual, and "hands on" instructions and guidance they give.

In Clinical Education

Therapy students are curious. They do want to learn and to study closely the patients they will be treating. The LNNB could give them an opportunity to study at least one diagnostic group in depth and observe the great variations involved. This might help students understand the futility of "diagnosis-treatment recipe cards." An example of how this might be done involves the thirty occupational therapy students in Dr. Dotty Weeks' research class at Indiana University who volunteered to assist with a pilot study. The study involved groups of Hooverwood nursing home residents suffering from various forms of dementing illnesses.

Groups of three students each were trained to administer and score *one* clinical scale of the LNNB. After practice on normals, the students were given the names of consenting residents who agreed to be tested by the students. In each student group, one student served as administrator and scorer, one as observer and scorer, while the third established rapport with the next resident to be tested. Test administrators and observers compared scoring following testing. The administrator then became the observer for the student establishing rapport and about to become the new test administrator for that resident. The observer then went on to establish rapport with the next resident. Thus the three students rotated the jobs of test administrator, observer and rapport-builder. After three to four testings, scores were identical.

Many students dropped out due to difficulty in establishing cooperative rapport sufficient to initiate testing. Those that remained were able to administer their one sub-test to 30–50 residents in approximately fifteen hours. These students reported gaining confidence in establishing rapport, test administration, and in themselves as therapists. They apparently learned first hand the differences and similarities of individuals with identical diagnoses. A portion of their neuroanatomy and neurology classes was reinforced. They received an opportunity to experience clinical research and they were of immense assistance in the project. Many residents looked forward to "talking with those nice students."

CONCLUSION

Therapists can use the LNNB to assist in mapping functional profiles of dementia victims and behavioral sequence and progression of the disease. Because our training and experiences are different from one another, and different from that of neuropsychologists and from social scientists, therapists of all kinds have the unique opportunity to find new associations, make discoveries and invent new solutions. To do this, we must be willing to go beyond the self-interest of our own disciplines, risk sharing our knowledge, have courage to seek assistance from those in other fields, and continually work to integrate new knowledge and skills into our practices and research. We can join the search for brain-behavior relationships, which is nothing more than a search for answers and solutions to such painful problems as dementia.

REFERENCES

American Psychiatric Association. (1980). *Diagnostic and statistical manual of mental disorders* (3rd ed.). Washington, DC: Author.

Botwinick, J. (1973). *Aging and behavior: A comprehensive integration of research findings.* New York: Springer Publishing Co.

Bischof, L. J. (1976). *Adult psychology.* New York: Harper & Row.

Bryant, E. T., Maruish, M. E., Golden, C. J. (1984). Validity of the Luria-Nebraska Neuropsychological Battery. *Journal of consulting and clinical psychology, 52,* 445–448.

Carnes, M. (1984). Diagnosis and management of dementia in the elderly. *Physical and Occupational Therapy in Geriatrics, 3*(4), 11–24.

Cattel, R. B. (1965). *The scientific analysis of personality.* Baltimore, MD: Penguin.

Cohen, D. (1982). Issues in psychological diagnosis and management of the cognitively impaired aged. In C. Eisdorfer & E. Fann (Eds.). *Treatment of psychopathology in aging.* New York: Springer Publishing Co.

Crosson, B., Warren, R. L. (1982). Use of the Luria-Nebraska Neuropsychological Battery in aphasia: A conceptual critique. *Journal of consulting and clinical psychology, 50,* 22–31.

Delis, D. C., & Kaplan, E. (1982). The assessment of aphasia with the Luria-Nebraska Neuropsychological Battery: A case critique. *Journal of consulting and clinical psychology, 50,* 32–39.

Drachman, D. A. (1980) An approach to the neurology of aging. In J. E. Birren & R. B. Sloane (Eds.). *Handbook of mental health and aging.* Englewood Cliffs, NJ: Prentice-Hall, Inc. pp. 508–509.

Eisdorfer, C. (1981). Management of the patient and family coping with dementing illness. *The journal of family practice. 12,* 831–837.

Eisdorfer, C., Cohen, D., & Preston, C. (1981). Behavioral and psychological therapies for the older patient with cognitive impairment. In N. E. Miller & G. D. Cohen (Eds.). *Clinical aspects of Alzheimer's Disease and senile dementia (Aging,* Vol. 15) New York: Raven Press.

Feinberg, I; Fein, G; Price, L. J.; Jernigan, T. L., & Floyd, T. C. (1980). Methodological and conceptual issues in the study of brain-behavior relations in the elderly. In L. W. Poon (Ed.). *Aging and the 1980's.* Washington DC: American Psychological Association.

Gillen, R. W., MacInnes, W. D., Golden, A. J. (1982, August). *Dementia and performance on the Luria-Nebraska Neuropsychological Battery.* Paper presented at the American Psychological Association Convention.

Gillen, R. W., Golden, C. J., & Eyde, D. R. (1982). Use of the Luria-Nebraska Neuropsychological Battery with elderly populations. *Clinical Gerontologist, 1*(2), 3–21.

Golden, C. J. (1981). *Diagnosis and rehabilitation in clinical neuropsychology.* Springfield, IL: Charles C. Thomas.

Golden, C. J., Ariel, R. N., McKay, S. E., Wilkening, G. N., Wolf, B. A., & MacInnes, W. D. (1982a). The Luria-Nebraska Neuropsychological Battery: Theoretical orientation and comment. *Journal of consulting and clinical psychology, 50,* 291–300.

Golden, C. J., Ariel, R. N., Moses, J. A., Wilkening, G. N., McKay, S. E., & MacInnes, W. D. (1982b). Analytic techniques in the interpretation of the Luria-Nebraska Neuropsychological Battery. *Journal of consulting and clinical psychology, 50,* 40–48.

Golden, C. J., Hammeke, T. A., & Purisch, A. D. (1983). *The Luria-Nebraska Neuropsychological Battery.* Los Angeles: Western Psychological Services.

Golden, C.J., Hammeke, T. A., Purisch, A. D., Berg, R. A., Moses, J. A., Newlin, D. B., Wilkening, G. H., & Puente, A. E. (1982c). *Item interpretation of the Luria-Nebraska Neuropsychological Battery.* Lincoln: University of Nebraska Press.

Goldstein, G. (1983). Normal aging and the concept of dementia. In Golden, C. J., & P. J. Vicente (Eds.) *Foundations of Clinical Neuropsychology.* New York: Plenum Press.

Hebb, D. O. (1945). *The Organization of Behavior* New York: John Wiley & Sons.

Hebb, D. O. (1966). *A Textbook of psychology.* Philadelphia, PA: W. B. Saunders Co.

Habot, B., & Libow, L. S. (1980). The interrelationship of mental and physical status and its assessment in the older adult: Mind-body interaction. In J. E. Birren & R. B. Sloane (Eds.), *Handbook of mental health and aging* (pp.698–730). Englewood, NJ: Prentice-Hall.

Hartlage, L. C., & DeFilippis, N. A. (1983). History of neuropsychological assessment. In C. J. Golden & P. J. Vicente (Eds.), *Foundations of clinical neuropsychology* (pp. 1–23). New York: Plenum Press.

Kane, R. A., Kane, R. L. (1983). *Assessing the elderly: A practical guide to measurement.* Lexington, MA: Lexington Books.

Kane, R. L., Sweet, J. J., Golden, C. J., Parsons, O. A., & Moses, J. A., (1981). Comparative diagnostic accuracy of the Halstead-Reitan and standardized Luria-Nebraska Neuropsychological Batteries in a mixed psychiatric and brain-damaged population. *Journal of consulting and clinical psychology, 49,* 484–485.

Kay, D. W. K., & Bergmann, K. (1980). Prevalence of dementia. In J. E. Birren & R. B. Sloane (Eds.), *Handbook of mental health and aging* (pp. 28–52). Englewood, NJ: Prentice-Hall.

Luria, A. R. (1969). *The origin and cerebral organization of man's conscious action.* Lecture to the XIX International Congress of Psychology. London, England.

MacInnes, W. D. (1981). *Healthy aging, brain structures and neuropsychological functioning.* Unpublished doctoral dissertation, University of Nebraska.

MacInnes, W. D. (1983a). Aging and dementia. In C. J. Golden, J. A. Moses, J. A. Coffman, W. A. Miller, & F. D. Strider (Eds.), *Clinical neuropsychology: Interface with neurologic and psychiatric disorders* (pp. 81–101). New York: Grune & Stratton.

MacInnes, W. D. (1983b). The use of the Luria-Nebraska Neuropsychological Battery in the diagnosis of dementia. *Bulletin, 2* (3), 7–9.

MacInnes, W. D., Franzen, M. D., Sawicki, R., Golden, C. J., Mahoney, P.,

McGill, J., Uhl, H. S. (1983, August). *Aging, neuropsychological functioning and brain density: Interrelationships.* Paper presented at the American Psychological Association Convention, Anaheim, CA.

MacInnes, W. D., Gillen, R. W., Golden, C. J., Graber, B., Cole, J., Uhl, H. S., & Greenhouse, A. H. (1983). Aging and performance on the Luria-Nebraska Neuropsychological Battery. *International journal of neurosciences, 19,* 179-190.

MacInnes, W. D., Golden, C. J., Gillen, R. W., Sawicki, R. F., Quaife, M., Uhl, H. S., & Greenhouse, A. J. (1984). Aging, regional cerebral blood flow and neuropsychological functioning. *Journal of the American Geriatric Society.*

MacInnes, W. D., & Quaife, M. (1982a, August). *Luria-Nebraska Neuropsychological Battery, regional cerebral blood flow and the elderly.* Paper presented at the American Psychological Association Convention, Washington, D. C.

MacInnes, W. D., Uhl, H. S., & Greenhouse, A. J. (1982b, August). *Healthy aging and performance on the Luria-Nebraska Neuropsychological Battery.* Paper presented at the American Psychological Association Convention, Washington, D. C.

Malloy, P. F., & Webster, J. S. (1981). Detecting mild brain impairment using the Luria-Nebraska Neuropsychological Battery. *Journal of consulting and clinical psychology, 49,* 768-770.

Miller, E. (1980). Cognitive assessment of the older adult. In J. E. Birren & R. B. Sloane (Eds.), *Handbook of mental health and aging* (pp. 520-536) Englewood Cliffs, NJ: Prentice-Hall.

Moses, J. A., Golden, C. J., Ariel, R. N., & Gustavson, J. L. (1983a). *Interpretation of the Luria-Nebraska Neuropsychological Battery: Vol. 1.* New York: Grune & Stratton.

Moses, J. A., Golden, C. J., Wilkening, G. N., McKay, S. E., & Ariel, R. N. (1983b). *Interpretation of the Luria-Nebraska Neuropsychological Battery: Vol. 2.* New York: Grune & Stratton.

National Institute of Health. (1981). *The dementias: Hope through research.* (NIH Publication No. 81-2252). Washington DC: US Government Printing Office.

National Institute on Aging. (1983, August). *Special Report on Aging, 1983.* (NIH Publication No. 83-2489). Washington, DC: US Department of Health and Human Services, Public Health Services.

National Institute on Aging Task Force. (1980). Senility reconsidered: Treatment for mental impairment in the elderly. *Journal of the American Medical Association, 244* (3), 259-263.

Ochsner, A. (1976). Aging. *Journal of the American Geriatrics Society, 24*(9), 385-393.

Patterson, R. L. (1982). *Overcoming deficits of aging: A behavioral approach.* New York: Plenum Press.

Post, F. (1980). Paranoid, schizophrenia-like and schizophrenic states in the aged. In J. E. Birren & R. B. Sloane (Eds.), *Handbook of mental health and aging* (pp. 594-595). Englewood Cliffs: Prentice-Hall.

Price, L. J., Fein, G., & Feinberg, I. (1980). Neuropsychological assessment of cognitive function in the elderly. In L. W. Poon (Ed.). *Aging in the 1980's: Psychological issues* (pp. 78-85). Washington DC: American Psychological Association.

Reisberg, B. (1981). *A guide to Alzheimer's Disease.* New York: The Free Press.

Reynolds, C. R. (1982). Determining statistically reliable strengths and weaknesses in the performance of single individuals on the Luria-Nebraska Neuropsychological Battery. *Journal of consulting and clinical psychology, 50,* 525-529.

Schaie, K. W. (1977). Quasi experimental research designs in the psychology of aging. In J. E. Birren & K. W. Schaie (Eds.), *Handbook of the psychology of aging* (pp. 692-723). New York: Van Nostrand-Reinhold.

Sloan, R. B. (1980). Organic brain syndrome, in J. E. Birren & R. B. Sloane (Eds.). *Handbook of mental health and aging* (pp. 570–594). Englewood Cliffs, Prentice-Hall, Inc.

Spiers, P. A. (1981). Have they come to praise Luria or to bury him? The Luria-Nebraska Battery controversy. *Journal of consulting and clinical psychology, 50,* 301–306.

Spinaris-Attrell, C. (1979). Comment: The dilemma of differential diagnosis: A reply to Ernst et al. *The Gerontologist, 19,* 526–529.

Spitzform, M. (1982). Normative data in the healthy elderly on the Luria-Nebraska Neuropsychological Battery. *Clinical Neuropsychology, 4,* 103–105.

Streib, G. F. (1983). The frail elderly: Research dilemmas and research opportunities. *The Gerontologist,* 23(1), 40–44.

Swendseid, G. (1982, August). *The neuropsychological functioning of an elderly nursing home population.* Paper presented at the American Psychological Association Convention, Washington, DC.

Zarit, S. H., Miller, N. E., Kahn, M. A., & Kahn, R. L. (1978). Brain function intellectual impairment and education in the aged. *Journal of the American Geriatrics Society,* 26 (2).

BOOK REVIEWS

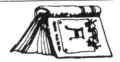

ALZHEIMER'S DISEASE HANDBOOK and STATE AND AREA AGENCY INSTRUCTIONAL GUIDE, Lindeman, D.; ALZHEIMER'S FAMILY SUPPORT GROUPS: A MANUAL FOR GROUP FACILITATORS, Middleton, L.; WORKING WITH FAMILIES OF DEMENTIA VICTIMS: A TREATMENT MANUAL, Zarit, S. (Four Volume Set) by *Department of Health and Human Services—Administration on Aging (available through Human Developmental Services Log # AoA - IM-84-39). Paper, 1984, no price available.*

These four volumes offer informational assistance for professionals who sponsor AoA family support groups for Alzheimer's disease victims.

Volume I, *Alzheimer's Disease Handbook,* contains four short chapters, a bibliography and a series of 14 appendices. Chapter one describes symptoms, diagnosis, causes and current treatment. The following chapter presents an overview of the psychosocial aspects of Alzheimer's. Chapter three lists institutional and community based resources, describes two treatment programs for Alzheimer's and gives addresses of long-term gerontology centers. The final chapter describes self-help and family support groups, as well as steps to establish your own group. The appendices offer exhaustive professional, behavioral and informational references.

Volume II, *State and Area Agency Instructional Guide,* serves as an accompanying instructional guide for using the *Alzheimer's Disease Book* (Vol. I.) It also offers a supplemental medical bibliography and a resource list for professionals in clinical and social service agencies.

Volume III, *Alzheimer's Family Support Groups,* guides professionals leading family support groups. Chapter one delineates Alzheimer's financial impact on American society and particularly the health care system. Chapter two first distinguishes between dementia, delirium, Alzheimer's disease and senility, then medically characterizes the disease. Alzheimer's disease has differentiating characteristics in its cause, course, and outcome. This chapter defines generic self-help and family support groups by their function and goals. Self-help groups offer mutual aid under a democratic construct whereby people determine how they view themselves, and how to obtain appropriate services to meet their needs. Family groups offer members or primary caregivers mutual assistance, encouragement, education, skills and support. As Chapter four states, people come to family support groups to understand and cope with common problems and concerns through shared experiences. This chapter describes how these support groups operate. A formal program at meetings may include knowledge, skills, techniques, resources and attitudes necessary for proper care and supervision of Alzheimer's victims. Chapter five outlines how to start a family support group. The professional must be knowledgeable about the disease; obtain the support of community services; and establish a medical ally (psychiatrist or physician). Ongoing planned activities include newsletters which keep families up-to-date on previous meeting's activities and details on upcoming meetings, securing speakers, publishing directories, and collecting information on Alzheimer's. Examples of newsletters, registration forms and program titles are included with references and suggested readings. Chapter six describes a model Family Support Group. The final chapter describes intervention through direct services (peer-support, casework services, counseling, and grief-support groups). It also explains the patient advocate role played by professionals. This chapter concludes with a categorical bibliography of both professional and lay oriented references.

Volume IV, *Working with Families of Dementia Victims: (A Treatment Manual),* addresses health-care professionals who directly intervene with patients and their families. It also serves as an instructional manual for gerontology students. This manual describes Alzheimer's, with other dementias and provides guidelines to indicate signs of dementia. Chapter four helps professionals plan appropriate intervention by determining current problems and resources and treating according to family member's preferences and values. A memory and behavior problems checklist and a quiz that allows a family to describe their feelings when caring for an Alzheimer's family member are helpful. Chapter five describes a successful intervention model that maintains the parent at home without overburdening caregivers. The following chapter compares one-to-one counseling, and family support group treatment techniques. Chapter seven discusses special problems in treatment, community interventions, and appropriate use of nursing homes. Chapter eight, a case study, depicts a professional's counseling sessions with a patient's wife over the long period of time of her husband's decline. The final chapter speculates future trends in management and treatment of dementia. The text concludes with a referential bibliography.

Of these four separate, yet interrelated volumes, Volume IV seems most useful for physical or occupational therapists. All four offer helpful information and guidelines for those allied medical professionals who work with the elderly. The large type, short paragraphs and chapters, plus its plain writing style makes comprehension quick and easy.

Paul I. Martin, RMT
Graduate Student
Music Therapy/Education
University of Iowa
Iowa City, IA

T - #0040 - 270225 - C0 - 216/138/8 [10] - CB - 9780866565561 - Gloss Lamination